BRAIN REFRAME

MOSAICA PRESS

אדם נפעל כפי פעולותיו

BRAIN REFRAME

THE 52 HABITS OF THE HIGHLY EFFECTIVE DIETER

BASYA KOVACS

ISBN: 978-1-961602-25-0

Published by Mosaica Press, Inc.
www.mosaicapress.com
info@mosaicapress.com

For more information: bkcoaching2023@gmail.com

Consult with your doctor before starting any weight loss program, particularly if you are pregnant, nursing, or have underlying medical conditions.

This book is dedicated to my husband

YEHUDA

and my five amazing children

SHLOMO SIM, SHIRA, HILLEL, ELI, AND AKIVA

Thank you to each of you. You are the lights of my life.
I am eternally grateful to Hashem
and more blessed than I can express in words.

ADVANCE PRAISE

TO THOSE OF YOU who have bought this book and are ready to take control of your eating, I want to wish you congratulations. As you may know from my podcasts and lectures, I often equate the discipline that is needed for spiritual growth to the discipline needed for exercise and eating right.

Bodies don't change instantly and neither does our spirituality. Eating right takes work and commitment, and so does our relationship with Hashem. Dieters will always have the *yetzer hara* telling them to quit or give in just this once, and so do spiritual growth seekers. People mess up on their diets, and people mess up spiritually.

The world below is simply a reflection of or a *mashal* for the world above. By taking the lessons in this book to heart, you will not only find a way—a template—for weight management that is attainable, sustainable, and which will make you healthier; you will find that if you apply the same tools spiritually, you will have a template for growth and connection with Hashem.

Focus on progress, not perfection. As Rebbe Nachman says, "God's ways are not like those of man. When a man makes a garment, he values it most when it is brand new. As it becomes worn and damaged, its value is reduced. But God began by creating an imperfect world. As it is constantly being improved, it becomes more precious to God."

With blessings for good health and success,
Gedale Fenster

THERE ARE MANY wellness coaches who know much about nutrition, exercise, and health. But rare is a wellness coach like Basya, who has a deep understanding of all of those areas, combined with a deep understanding of people, and specifically the person sitting in front of her.

She meets her clients where they are at, in their health, in their mindset, and in their own personal goals. She has the ability to empathize, yet leads clients to their goals in a recipe for success—emotionally and physically.

Debbie Selengut, kallah teacher, Passaic, New Jersey

WHEN I SIGNED up to work with Basya, I was skeptical. I figured it was just another diet, more of the same. I wish you could hear my passion as I say the next few words: There is something unique about Basya's approach! Much of what I learned from working with Basya was life changing and mind blowing. What is obvious to her should have been obvious to me all my life. But it wasn't.

Basya's commitment to the truth and her determination to help people succeed is quite impressive. I am excited that Basya will be able to help you and many others through this breakthrough writing, *Brain Reframe*!

Happy reading!

Shifi Lieberman, LMFT
www.ShifiLieberman.com

RABBI DOVID GOLDWASSER הרב דוד גאלדוואסער

Rosh Chodesh Cheshvan, 5784

והנה כתוב בספר ראשית חכמה:
בעיניו יראה כונות האכילה אשר שוו בשעוריהן עם הקרבנות.
אשרי ילוד אשה אשר ידו משגת להיות בונה בשמים עליותיו על ידי אכילותיו
ובלב שיכון לבו לשמים ויעשה הדברים כדת וכהלכה
(פלא יועץ)

The *Sefer Reishis Chachmah* states that if one partakes of his food with the proper *kavanah* it is as if he offered a *korban* in the *Bais HaMikdash*. Blessed is mortal man who is able to build *aliyos* in *Shamayim* merely by consuming his food for the sake of Heaven.

Mrs. Basya Kovacs has written an important work, entitled *Brain Reframe*. It is dedicated to helping people who struggle with issues of healthy eating, dieting and body image. She draws on her considerable experience as a therapist and counselor. She provides the reader with real-life case histories, advice on healthy eating, and useful nutritional information.
Mrs. Kovacs engages the reader with an easygoing yet direct approach to a most challenging topic.

I believe that Basya Kovacs' book will be a great benefit and support to those who are trying to navigate the complexities of dieting and proper nutrition.

I wish the author much continued *hatzlacha* in her work as a therapist and guide to the community. May she be *zoche* to be counted among the מצדיקי הרבים שצדקתם עומדת לעד.

המצפה לישועה,
Rabbi Dovid Goldwasser

1336 EAST 21ST STREET · BROOKLYN, NY 11210 · TEL. 718-339-4582 / STUDY 718-677-3712

Have your cake and eat it, too.

Old English Proverb

TABLE OF CONTENTS

PREFACE

I BELIEVE THAT I am uniquely qualified to write this book, not so much because of my fourteen years of working with clients and helping them lose weight. That part is true. But my main qualification is that I am a former fat girl who has mastered the art of truly having it all. I say "fat" not as an insult, but as a simple fact. I have figured out how to eat what I love, eat plenty of it, and still maintain a healthy (okay, thin) figure. I love food. I love to eat. Also, I hate rules and I am not a particularly disciplined person. And my passion in life is to share what I have learned with you so that you and your relationship with food can live happily ever after.

Let me tell you a little about myself, my journey, and how I got to where I am today. When I was a kid, I was pretty carefree. My earliest memories are mostly happy ones, and my childhood was unencumbered. A free spirit, I loved nature, sports, swimming, and reading. I could lose myself for hours in books, and I was a bright and happy kid.

Oh—and eating. I loved to eat. Family folklore has it that I used to sleep talk and say the words "sweet potato" when I was a year old. Apparently, I hadn't yet developed my current, ever-so-much-more sophisticated taste for chocolate. My mother also claims that people used to comment that I should be bounced down the street rather than walked, referencing my plump, roundish shape. And I distinctly recollect asking for a refrigerator full of food one year for an afikoman present, which I did not get, and a bag of gum lollipops a different year, which I did. My brothers received a 10-speed bike.

As I grew older, I also grew taller, like really tall. And I thinned out as I stretched. I am currently five foot, nine inches, and I grew to be almost this height by the time I was in seventh grade. This is where my story really begins, because that is when I started feeling self-conscious about my height. By the time I was in seventh or eighth grade, I wasn't just the tallest kid in the class, but the tallest person in the school, including teachers and even principals.

My love for food hadn't affected my weight just yet, but regardless, I felt pretty uncomfortable in my skin. I didn't know how to express it at the time, but looking back, my body image issues began around puberty. My mother, also five foot, nine inches, was—and still is—beautiful, confident, and graceful. I didn't know how to express my discomfort to her, didn't have the right words, or even the self-awareness of what was bothering me.

What does this have to do with my weight? Nothing at first. I was still super athletic and, like I said, I was growing and stretching, so I remained thin. My first memory of feeling fat was at the age of eleven. I remember going to a cousin's bar mitzvah out on Long Island. I flew in from Chicago with a couple of family members and had never been to such a high-end event before. I have a distinct recollection of being pulled by the sheer abundance of food, gorging on it, and then feeling awful later that night. I recall lying on my grandmother's spare foldaway cot, crying to my mother that I felt fat. This was probably the first time that I expressed being uncomfortable in my body, but it was kind of a one-time thing.

I remained athletic, swimming four to five times a week and playing ball with my friends. This is where I felt the most alive, and the most at ease. But the rest of the time, I struggled. I couldn't find normal clothes and couldn't relate to the lessons my teachers taught about how we, as women, are all princesses. I didn't feel like a princess. I felt overgrown and awkward. I couldn't buy pretty shoes because they looked monstrous and odd, so I stuck to high-top sneakers that made my feet feel smaller, at least in my eyes. I couldn't buy the latest-style clothes, because they didn't fit me right and didn't cover my knees. I couldn't even buy normal knee socks that my private school required, because they reached nowhere near my knees, so my mother would buy me long black socks that were made for men. Awkward.

By the end of eighth grade, I finally stopped growing. Phew! I also stopped swimming as much and couldn't spend hours and hours playing ball like I did in elementary school, and that's when the real trouble started. I stopped growing and slowed down the athletics, but I kept on eating. By the time I was in tenth grade, I weighed almost thirty pounds more than I had in eighth grade and graduated from awkward to distinctly uncomfortable.

I couldn't fit into my clothes and did not fit in with my friends. I just wanted to be normal. And so, in tenth grade, I went on my very first diet.

This set off a cycle of attempting various diets, which all had one thing in common. They didn't work. Well, they worked at first, but each one left me fatter and more uncomfortable than the one before. (Sound familiar?)

Fortunately, I met my husband when I was twenty years old, and his eating habits had a tremendous impact on mine. I learned the art of moderation. I learned that vegetables are actually delicious. He also taught me the value of self-care. And he unconditionally loved me. I had five children in seven years, and my body shape shifted almost seasonally, and he loved me at every size. I finally felt like a princess.

Slowly, over time, my new habits took hold, and by the time I had my last two children (twins!), I truly felt that my new habits were a part of me. My twins are eleven now, and when I lost the baby weight, I knew I was losing weight for the last time. I have kept my weight off since then.

More recently, I had the good fortune of coming across the teachings of Rebbe Nachman of Breslov through the venerable Gedale Fenster. His teachings had a tremendous influence on my worldview, and I developed an entirely new perspective on discomfort, pain, and challenges. These teachings helped me develop a new level of consciousness, as I began to see challenges, including my relationship with food, as opportunities for growth and connection with Hashem. You will notice Rebbe Nachman's influence throughout the book, and my prayer is that you will benefit from this added dimension.

I wrote this book because I feel like I have found the secret to success and I want to share it with as many people as I can, so that they can enjoy their food and feel great in their bodies. You can have it all. You can have your cake and eat it, too. Just not too much and not every day.

Basya Kovacs
January 2024

ACKNOWLEDGMENTS

THIS BOOK is the end result of years of working with hundreds if not thousands of clients of all ages and backgrounds. I want to start by thanking you, my clients, for teaching me everything I know, and allowing me to be your coach. You have given me more than any schooling can provide. You have entrusted me with your deepest thoughts and experiences, taught me what works and what doesn't, and given me precious insight that I in turn can share with others. I am in awe of the incredible changes that you have undergone, the mindset shifts that you have made that have impacted your entire lives, and most of all I am amazed at your determination to take ownership of your destiny. Thank you for allowing me to be on this journey with you.

I also want to acknowledge all the people who supported me from the very beginning: Tanya Rosen, thank you for the opportunity to make a difference in so many people's lives. Aliza W. and Gitty L., thank you for believing in this book when it was still in its very rough stages. Tova T. and Doni R., thank you for cheering me on and helping me get to the finish line. Naomi J., thank you for showing me what is possible, and for guiding me on this journey. Solomon H., you made sure this book stayed funny—your specialty—thank you! Shavy W., D.B., and Devorah, thank you for standing by my side when things got challenging. And those of you who asked that your names be left out, I am honoring your request, but please know that I am forever grateful to you.

To my two mentors, Sunny Levi and Gedale Fenster, I am forever indebted to you. Sunny, from you I learned to thank Hashem for the sunshine and the rain. And Gedale, from you I learned what my mission on this earth is—to grow even though it might not always feel good. The daily *hisbodedus* and daily classes have changed my entire outlook on life, and my hope is that I am *zocheh* to continue to internalize your message, and, if I am worthy, pass my inspiration to others.

To the incredible Mosaica team, who patiently brought this book into fruition: Your dedication, professionalism, and unwavering support throughout every step of the publishing process has been phenomenal. From conceptualizing and crystallizing the ideas in this book to editing and re-editing, as well as in the meticulous design work, your patience and commitment to excellence was constant. I feel so blessed to have collaborated with such a talented group of professionals. You not only improved the content of this book but also made the journey toward publication a positive and enjoyable experience. Thank you for your endless support, professional expertise, and for truly turning my vision into a reality. I am forever grateful.

To my incredible parents: Thank you for being my role models. You have taught me what it means to give and to love without expecting anything in return. You have taught me to live with integrity and pure faith, yet never judge anyone else. You have stood by my side through every step of this amazing learning experience called life. I am so grateful and so extremely blessed.

To Yehuda, my knight in shining armor: I don't have the right words to express my appreciation for you. You have been my support, my confidant, my rock and my partner in every sense of the word. Thank you for accepting me for who I am, and for always knowing just what I need, whether its space, time, support, or a nap! They don't make them quite like you. You are my hero.

To Shlomo Simcha, Shira, Hillel, Eli, and Akiva: I am so lucky to be your mother. Each of you is so different, and each of you makes me so proud. I love watching you grow into amazing mini adults. You have rock-solid integrity, kindness, grace, and loyalty. You care about the feelings of others and value what's important—Hashem, family, and friendships. You are so unspoiled, and you make even the simplest things fun. Being your mom is my greatest honor. You have been cheering me on for years, and I thank Hashem for each of you every single day.

Finally, I want to thank Hashem for allowing me to bring this book to fruition. I am humbled by all the blessings You shower upon me, and my only hope is that You allow me to continue to make an impact on the lives of others. I will do my best to be worthy of Your abundant kindness.

INTRODUCTION

THE D WORD

There once was a woman named Leah (name is fictional, although I'm sure this scenario definitely happened at least once to a woman named Leah), who decided she wanted to lose weight, so she did what all self-respecting Americans do—she went on a diet. She chose the most popular diet that was all the rage at that time, which involved some pseudoscience and touted extreme results such as twenty pounds in twenty minutes, as long as you stand on one foot and eat carbs only between the minutes of 8:11 and 8:17 every day—you know the type of diet I'm talking about.

Anyway, after following the diet religiously for some time, she managed to bamboozle off fourteen pounds in about a month. Pleased with her results, she promptly went off the diet. Understandably, she missed her normal food. She then proceeded to gain twenty-two pounds in two months, which should shock none of you, and decided it was time to go back on that diet—also predictable.

Only this time, she lost eleven pounds, and it took her almost three months because, honestly, she didn't quite have it in her to stick to the diet the way she had originally. After losing eleven pounds, she felt frustrated, so she did what all self-respecting American dieters do—she made her way over to a brand-new, sparkly diet, glittering with the promise of ten pounds in ten days, and, of course, this one promised that she would keep it off forever. She obviously did not. She subsequently tried another diet that worked until it didn't and then another, which also worked until it didn't.

Each round of abusing her body, eating food she hated, and ultimately failing and gaining the weight back plus interest was more and more demoralizing and discouraging, and soon Leah's weight ballooned to over two hundred pounds.

By now, Leah decided her only recourse was to explore surgical options. She wasn't too excited about weight loss surgery because of the obvious risks involved, but she was feeling so defeated by the process and so overwhelmed with the amount of weight she had to lose that she just wanted to be done with her weight once and for all. Six months later, she went under the knife, hopeful that she would finally lose weight for good. She went through the surgery and after a year of losing like a champ, she stopped losing. And then she started to gain weight back. And with terror, she realized that she was heading right back to where she started.

Does any part of this cycle sound even vaguely familiar? The endless cycle of losing quickly, gaining back with interest, finding a new miracle, rinse, and repeat, is pretty common in our dieting culture. The good news is that it really doesn't have to be this way. We can end this cycle—all you need to do is lend me your brain for a year, so we can rewire some of your old thought processes, deeply ingrained beliefs, and habits and end this nonsense once and for all, for real this time. Sounds easy enough, right? Wrong. It takes some work to rewire the brain, but it can be done.

Let's start by defining the word "diet"—according to me. While most people think of the word "diet" as a way of losing weight, often by restricting food groups or calories, I define it as the parameters and rules you choose to eat by in order to achieve your health and wellness goals. For example, if I have celiac disease, I may go on a gluten-free diet, and if I am an Orthodox Jew, I may keep a kosher diet. Therefore, while I don't like the word "diet" because of its negative connotations, I actually think that everyone should follow a diet. Meaning to say that everyone should have systems and guidelines in place for how they eat, instead of just eating whatever, and whenever.

This means that whether you are morbidly obese, severely underweight, or chilling comfortably at your goal weight, you should still be on a diet. Which diet, you ask? Ah. We will get to that soon. But if we are defining the word "diet" as a food-intake management system, we should all be on diets forever. I hope I didn't lose you all there. By understanding that I need to be on a diet forever, I will no longer see dieting as a punitive short-term weight loss project, but, rather, as a long-term system of eating in order to reach and maintain my health and wellness goals, while taking my actual life into account.

There—I said it. It can't just be a diet; it needs to be a lifestyle change! I know, it's a cliché, as all diet books promise a lifestyle plan. But realistically, they fail to deliver. They proceed to espouse the latest fad or miracle, tell you exactly what to eat and what not to eat for twenty to thirty pages, and then finish off with one hundred pages of complex recipes that no one ever uses. This book is not that. This is a book about rewiring our brains, changing our relationship with food, and, ultimately, changing our relationship with ourselves in the process. Also, this book is kind of funny—I try not to take myself too seriously.

A WORD ON BODY POSITIVITY

Let's talk about body positivity for a minute. According to the website verywellmind.com, "body positivity" refers to the assertion that all people deserve to have a positive body image, regardless of how society and popular culture view ideal shape, size, and appearance.

Some of the goals of the body positivity movement:

- Challenging how society views the body.
- Promoting the acceptance of all bodies.
- Helping people build confidence and acceptance of their own bodies.
- Addressing unrealistic body standards.

Body positivity is not just about challenging how society views people based upon their physical size and shape, however. It also recognizes that judgments are often made based on race, gender, sexuality, and disability.

Body positivity also aims to help people understand how popular media messages contribute to the relationship that people have with their bodies, including how they feel about food, exercise, clothing, health, identity, and self-care.

By better understanding the effect that such influences have, the hope is that people can develop a healthier and more realistic relationship with their bodies.

I am all for body positivity. This book was not written to tell you how to look or how to feel about your body. This book isn't designed to set your goals for you or to pressure you into fitting into someone else's beauty or health paradigm. This book was written for you to help you reach your weight and health goals. If you are happy and healthy and love your body, God bless you—you may want to lend this book to a friend. But if you appreciate the benefits of having a roadmap for the way you eat, and if you want to add an element of structure to your eating habits that will likely affect discipline in all aspects of your life, this book is for you.

ABOUT THIS BOOK

This book is titled *Brain Reframe: The 52 Habits of Highly Effective Dieters*. While some of the chapters discuss habits in the traditional sense, such as keeping a food log or making sure your food is prepared in advance, you'll find that many of the chapters discuss new and different ways of thinking about the weight loss process. While we tend to think of habits as actions, such as cracking our knuckles (mindless habit) or brushing our teeth (mindful habit), we tend to forget that our thoughts are actually habits, too.

Did you ever realize that most of the thoughts that we have each day are thoughts we've already had before?

We have an internal running commentary that goes on throughout the day, almost like a psychotic roommate that is endlessly just there, narrating in the background.

Picture this scene:

It's 4:00 p.m. and you are headed to your kids' school for a carpool pickup.

"I have to get to my kids' school on time so that I am not the last mom there again...Hey, that car is the same as my car...I wonder if I turned the stove off before I left home...Wow, that's an interesting outfit choice that the teacher is wearing...Why is this seat so uncomfortable?...I should really get my car cleaned...Maybe I'll have the kids clean it...Oh good, there's another mom pulling up behind me...God bless her..."

On and on, the running commentary goes. None of these thoughts are particularly new or interesting. In fact, when we do have a brand-new thought or hear an idea that really stops and gets us thinking, it's actually really exciting.

The thing about our thoughts is that our thoughts are what create our feelings.

Let's go back to our commentary above:

"I have to get to my kids' school on time so that I am not the last mom there again." *Tension starts to set into your jaw.*

"Hey, that car is the same as my car!" *A jolt of pleasure when you realize that you like the car that you are looking at and you have the same one.*

"I wonder if I turned the stove off before I left home." *You might get an uncomfortable feeling of nerves in your stomach.*

"Wow, that's an interesting outfit choice that the teacher is wearing." *A flash of pride along with another small flash of pleasure when you compare your fine taste in clothes to the teacher's rather lacking sense of style.*

"Why is this seat so uncomfortable?" *Annoyance creeps in.*

"I should really get my car cleaned." *You might be a bit aggravated, and the tightness in your chest intensifies because the car never seems to stay clean.*

"Maybe I'll have the kids clean it." *Your body relaxes slightly.*

"Oh good, there's another mom pulling up behind me...God bless her!" *Your tension loosens, and you breathe more freely.*

So, you see—while our thoughts may be automatic, they actually affect how we feel emotionally and physically throughout the day. And even more importantly, our feelings affect our behavior. This is not news to any of us.

Back to our carpool scene. If I show up tense, I might be more likely to yell at my kids for kicking the seat on the way home. If I am calm and relaxed, I will probably be the better, more tolerant version of myself.

If our thoughts affect our feelings, and our feelings affect our behaviors, then it is actually quite critical that we don't allow our thoughts to run wild, on autopilot.

The good news is that if having the same thought over and over again creates a "thinking habit," then by thinking about things differently over and over again, we can create a new thinking habit.

And if the old way of thinking was causing feelings and behaviors that sabotaged our eating habits, then developing new and more-helpful thought patterns will automatically establish new, more helpful behavior patterns.

Let's take a typical thought pattern to which we can all relate. Say you have been sticking to your food plan religiously (for the thousandth time), and you find yourself super stressed. You fight it for a bit, but before you know it, you end up fist deep in a bag of chips. The old thought pattern may have said, "Well, I have messed up my diet anyway, so I might as well just finish this bag of chips and start again tomorrow." We will refer to this as "thought pattern A." We have all had this thought at some point or another—probably without even thinking about it. It literally just shows up, gets a pass, and we behave accordingly.

Imagine if you replaced that thought with something more helpful to your waistline, which we will refer to as "thought pattern B," such as, "If I stop eating these chips now, I will save myself from the seven hundred calories left in the bag. And while my weight loss might be slightly affected by the three hundred calories I just consumed, I can still get right back on track and the effect will be minimal. I'm going to do this differently this time."

Thought pattern A starts with a black-and-white thought: "I can't be perfect today, so I might as well give up and try again some other time." This thought brings along feelings of disappointment about not having a perfect day, and possibly frustration, having been down this road before. The disappointment is mollified by reassuring yourself that you'll start again tomorrow, and with lightning speed, the bag of chips is gone.

Thought pattern B allows us to feel hopeful and empowered. While we may not trust the feeling just yet, because it is new, it allows us to put down the chips and walk away.

It's that simple: new thought = new feeling = new behavior.

This is actually the therapeutic model upon which cognitive behavioral therapy, also known as CBT, is based. It is also aligned with the teachings of Rebbe Nachman.

By taking the time to really focus on each of these chapters, you will train yourself to stop your automatic thoughts in their tracks and rethink them. Do this often enough, and these thoughts become automatic—aka habits.

Lend me your brain for a year, and together we will develop the fifty-two habits of the highly effective dieter.

Please note: This book is written in what may or may not be a logical order. Feel free to spend as much (or as little) time as you need on each chapter. Feel free to work on a few of the habits at once. Please remember that developing new thoughts takes time. And practice. While this is divided up into fifty-two chapters, as in one new habit per week, understand that this is completely arbitrary. This is your brain. Set your pace as you see fit.

PART I

LOSING THE WEIGHT

1

FIND YOUR WHY

WE ALL EMBARK on our weight loss journeys for different reasons. Just kidding. Most of us undertake this process for several major reasons. First, we want to look better. Yup. I said it. The main reason most people actually start dieting is to look more attractive. We also do this for our health, to feel better in our clothes, to be good role models for those around us, and to feel more in control of our food intake, even if our weight is not a major problem. There are other reasons as well, but those are the main reasons I hear about in my private practice, and after working with over five thousand clients, I believe this pretty much sums it up.

However, sometimes we get lost on the way. We forget that there are many reasons why we choose to change our lifestyle, and it becomes all about the numbers on the scale moving to the left, assuming you are using an archaic doctor's scale like I do. (If you want to know why I choose that over a digital scale, email me—I don't want to have this on the record.) Anyway, back to my point. People get so stuck on the numbers, that when they don't lose fast enough, they tend to get frustrated and ultimately drift off their plan. If we could just keep our eye on the entire picture and remind ourselves why we wanted this in the first place, aside from just weight loss, we would be much more resilient when faced with minimal results or slower-than-expected weight loss. We also wouldn't quit quite as easily.

Let me tell you the story about one of my clients, Mike. Mike came into my office with about fifteen pounds to lose. After a few weeks, I realized he wasn't making much progress; every week was another story about why he couldn't stay on plan. I finally asked him directly, "Do you actually want to lose weight? Because you're not significantly overweight, and you don't have any health conditions—and you don't seem that motivated to stick to your plan." He answered, "To tell you the truth, I'm mostly here for my wife. She wants me to lose the extra weight, but I personally don't care that much."

Well, I thought to myself, *this will never do*.

I pressed him again, "Is there anything in this for you?" After considering the question for a bit, he began hesitantly, "Well, I don't want to eat everything I see—I want to be more disciplined and controlled, rather than just pulled wherever my mood or appetite takes me. And I *am* noticing that my weight is slowly creeping up, so I would like to nip that in the bud."

That's what I needed to hear. And that was what he needed to realize. Without knowing his "why" with absolute clarity, there would be no consistency and no motivation. And the opposite is for sure true. If you have a clear picture of why you want to do this, the work will seem less difficult.

Make a list of the reasons you will personally benefit from being disciplined about your food, and refer to this list regularly—at least twice a day. You see, when we first get started with our weight loss program, we are firing on all cylinders. We are hyper-focused, and our food plan takes front-and-center stage. But as life comes at us, which it always does, we tend to drift back to our old habits, and the food plan takes a back seat at best, or, sometimes, no seat at all.

Now, ideally, you would be able to conjure up your reasons just at the very moment that the chocolate chip cookie is making its way from your hand into your mouth. Boom. You are remotivated, and the cookie drops to the floor with a thud. Although that level of awareness is definitely possible (and we'll get there), for now just make a habit of reading the reasons you want to lose weight out loud, twice a day. If you develop this habit, which takes less time than it takes to floss (also a good habit, by the way), your motivation will never be far from the front of your mind.

Now, some of you will just keep reading, thinking, "I already know why I want to lose weight or stick to my plan—I don't need to write it down." Others will like the idea of writing it down and reading it out loud, but it will remain just that—a great idea in theory. But some of you will actually write your mission statement down and develop the habit of reading it out loud twice a day, maybe even while flossing. Those of you in the third category will be rewiring your brain, allowing your goals and dreams to remain front and center, possibly even being handy enough to pop right into your brain just as the cookie is about to enter your mouth. It's up to you to choose which category of people you wish to belong to.

BRAIN DRAIN

I don't know why I'm not as motivated anymore!

BRAIN RETRAIN

I can't expect to always stay motivated. But I can and will remotivate myself regularly. When I am about to quit, I will remember why I started.

2

GOALS

CLIENTS OFTEN ASK ME what their goal should be. They whip out the BMI chart and eagerly place their fingers at various points on the paper and try to determine if they are obese or merely overweight, all the while secretly despairing about the daunting task that lies ahead. Don't fret. The BMI chart doesn't mean much and, oftentimes, doesn't tell the whole picture. You have my permission to toss the BMI chart in the trash. That's right. Trash.

To determine your goal weight, there are only three factors that matter, in my opinion.

Choose a goal that is sustainable via normal, realistic eating habits. Don't choose a number that you once reached when you were starving yourself before your daughter's wedding, or the weight you once reached when you were nineteen, or when you had that horrible (but, let's be honest, kind of delightful) stomach virus that caused you to shed nine pounds in the course of three days.

Make sure that you will be healthy at the goal you choose. Healthy, meaning that your doctor isn't concerned about your A1C, blood pressure, cholesterol, or joints. The numbers tell the story better than the BMI chart ever will.

Choose a goal that feels great for you. It's your body—you are the one who lives inside it, and you are the one who needs to love it—no chart should determine this for you.

That's it. To review, choose a weight that is sustainable, healthy, and makes you feel great. The rest really doesn't matter. I have plenty of clients who fall into the overweight category on the BMI chart but have learned to ignore that chart for the sake of their sanity—you can feel free to do the same.

And the opposite is true as well. I've had too many instances where clients kept pushing the envelope, cutting food from their plan every time they hit a plateau, in order to reach some abstract goal that wasn't sustainable or even necessary. And then, feeling hungry and deprived, they ended up quitting, going back to their old eating habits, and gaining the weight back. Had they chosen a realistic goal, they would have been able to sustain their weight loss.

A word about maintenance—creating a maintenance plan for once you hit that plateau is critical. See the last few chapters for advice on maintenance—it's arguably the most important part of the book.

Once you choose your goal, assume you'll lose about a pound a week, on average, until you get there. If you have twenty-five pounds to lose, it'll take about half a year to lose it, and if you have fifty pounds to lose, give it a year. This may sound like a long time, but in the scheme of things, a year isn't that long. And while we all long for the quick fix, time is actually our friend. While our bodies can drop weight faster, our brains need time and practice in order to rewire the old thought patterns and habits—hence, the title of this book.

Don't rush the process—90 percent of dieters who lose more than 20 percent of their body weight gain it back within the year—mostly because they lose too quickly, don't give this process the time it needs to rewire their thinking patterns and behaviors, and, therefore, go right back to their old habits...and weight.

BRAIN DRAIN

According to my doctor and the BMI chart, I have so much to lose—I'll never get there.

BRAIN RETRAIN

I will choose a healthy, sustainable goal to reach at which I'll feel great. And I'll take it five pounds at a time. There is no rush.

3
FOREVER

NOW, IT'S TIME for you to create your diet. I am using the word "diet" the way we now understand it, which means a framework as well as a structured system that you choose, in order to manage your weight. That's right—you choose.

I have been in practice for over thirteen years, and what I have found is that most of my clients know what they need to do in order to lose weight. They just need help doing it. And despite trying all the various fad diets out there, most of my clients know that those only work in the short term. They jump from one diet fad to the next in the desperate hope that this new shiny diet will be the answer to their woes, without realizing that the answer is simple. Find something that is realistic and sustainable. And then develop the discipline needed to sustain it.

I'll give you a few more guidelines as to what has worked for many of my clients, but in the end, it's really about you.

Make sure you aren't cutting out any full food groups. If you are, you are guaranteed to only be able to stay on your diet for the short term. And as soon as you go off your plan, you will go back to those foods with a vengeance. (Let's all be honest here—we're talking about carbs.) I'm sure you have been down that road.

Don't confuse health and weight loss. People can gain weight on fruits, nuts, avocados, and salmon the same way that they can gain weight on pizza and chocolate. Too much food is too much food. Make sure that you incorporate realistic portion sizes into your plan.

On the other hand, nutritious food is more filling. Making healthy choices allows you to stay on track by keeping your blood sugar stable and reducing cravings. Make sure to include whole grains and veggies even though I just said in the previous paragraph that health and weight loss are mutually exclusive.

Eat regularly throughout the day. Going too long without food slows the metabolism and usually causes double trouble later on in the day. I recommend that my clients eat every two to three hours, to avoid the all-too-familiar 4:00 p.m. adult meltdown.

Incorporate fun. If you love pizza, have some. Just not only. If you love chocolate, incorporate it into your plan—just not every day. (Okay, fine, every day, but just a little.) Depriving yourself of the foods you love is a temporary, unsustainable punishment. Don't do it. And don't see this as a failure or something that is better off avoided—see it as part of Plan A.

Test and tweak. Using the above tips, write out a plan for yourself, including the foods that you want to be eating, the portion sizes that you feel will allow you to be satisfied while still losing weight, and the schedule to which you would like to stick. Make sure you write a plan for Erev Shabbos and Shabbos as well, and don't forget to work in the fun stuff.

Weigh yourself at the beginning of the week, and again a week later—same time and same place. If you lost between one and three pounds, you are on the right track. If you lost less than a pound, the pace may be a bit slow and frustrating for you, so try to determine where you can cut back slightly without leaving yourself feeling deprived and vulnerable. If you lost more than three pounds (or, after the first week, more than two pounds), you may be eating too little. Add some food in a systematic way so that you don't lose too quickly; while losing fast seems exciting, it usually backfires.

If you aren't sure if your plan will work, you can try it for a week, track your food on a food log (more on that later), and see how you do. If you lose a pound or two—keep at it. If you don't, pare it down a little and try again. You've got this.

Reminder—the only plans that I don't recommend are plans that either cut food groups out completely, allow too little food, or don't include your favorite foods. These types of plans are temporary measures, and we are so over that. This time we're doing this for real. Ready? Let's do this.

BRAIN DRAIN

That's it, I'm going vegan/paleo/keto/
gluten-free/crazy.

BRAIN RETRAIN

I am ready to try something actually sustainable—
something as close to my regular way of eating
as possible.

4

THE TIME IS NOW

I HAD BEEN working with a client, Rochel, for several months, and after seeing the progress she had made, her husband, Michael, decided to join the fun as well. After about a week on plan, I received the following text message from Rochel:

"My husband has been doing very well with his plan this past week, and he already lost three pounds. However, over Shabbos he struggled. And now, we have a family wedding, and then it is going to be Chanukah, and in a few weeks, he is scheduled to travel for work. Michael is feeling a bit overwhelmed by all these challenges and is wondering if we should pause the diet until February because he won't be traveling again until April."

While I hear her concerns, I strongly disagree with her premise, as I believe that it is quite shortsighted. Say her husband—or the average dieter for that matter—has thirty to fifty pounds to lose. Say he loses at a pace of one and a half to two pounds per week. This means he will need to stick to a disciplined food plan for approximately six months. This isn't even factoring maintenance into the equation. While April 1st may seem like a more convenient time to start dieting, there is no way her husband, or anyone, will have a six-month stretch to focus on nothing but dieting.

After Chanukah comes winter break. And then, there are *Shabbosim*, work events, and then, along comes summer. Summer brings with it a lack of routine, barbecues, and those long Motzaei Shabbos nights. After summer comes back-to-school and, shortly afterward, Thanksgiving, and then it's Chanukah again. There never was, and never will be, an "easy" six-month stretch to get into a routine. Additionally, the fact that Michael was discouraged by his first Shabbos on the plan, which comes *every week*, confirms for me that the "right time" to diet may never actually arrive.

Ultimately, we need to consider our plan to be a lifestyle. Six months is only the first step in a lifetime of eating on plan *despite* the challenges that come our way. *Yamim Tovim*, travel, restaurant meals, and family gatherings are all manageable on your plan, as long as you are committed. Because your plan factors in real life; it is not a quick fix.

My response to the concerned wife is the same as what I tell all my clients. Do not wait until the perfect time to start. There may be a perfect week or two, which will fool you into thinking that the right time has arrived, but there is *never* a stretch of six months of quietness, and that is a blessing. We *want* our lives to be rich and full. And we *want* to experience all that while still sticking to a disciplined food plan that allows us to enjoy and participate without overeating and gaining weight. We need to stop looking at every event or occasion as a reason to lose sight of our goals. If we are determined enough and committed enough and our plan is realistic enough, we can stay on track through it all.

So, if you are waiting until after Shabbos, or Sukkos, or Chanukah, or the move, or until the kids get settled in camp to start eating right, please reconsider. The time to start is *now*.

BRAIN DRAIN

I will wait until after Yom Tov to get started because then I will really be able to stick to my plan.

BRAIN RETRAIN

Waiting for the perfect time to diet is an illusion that allows me to keep eating poorly. There is never a good time to diet perfectly, but I can start now with a realistic food plan that I can stick to through anything that life throws my way.

5

BUT SERIOUSLY, WHAT SHOULD I EAT?

WARNING: If you already have a food plan that works for you and takes into consideration all of the "forever" guidelines from the previous chapter, please feel free to skip this chapter. However, if you are overwhelmed by the endless diet trends and fads and find yourself not knowing where to start, I'm going to give you some guidelines for what to eat, when to eat, and how much to eat. Again, I promised you that this book is not another diet book, so I'm trying to hold myself to that, but I don't want to leave you hanging if you could use a bit of extra guidance. If something in the next few chapters doesn't speak to you, please don't do it.

The reason pretty much every diet out there fails is not only because they are usually too restrictive or because they cut out major food groups (such as chocolate), or even because they are misguided. They fail because, despite what they may be promising, they are not the experts. Well, they may be the experts on food, but you are the expert on you.

You know what foods you love and what foods you hate. You know which foods are triggering and which ones are satisfying. You know which foods are too costly or too difficult to prepare, what times of the day or the week are the most challenging, and where you are most likely to derail. It is not likely that any one specific plan is going to be the final frontier. But that doesn't mean you shouldn't have a plan. It just means that you should be the designer of your plan, and your plan should be a living, breathing document, not dissimilar to the US Constitution, which is amended and molded (for better or for worse) to accommodate the ever-changing landscape of life.

The goal of this chapter will be to allow you to create a weight loss plan that is practical, sustainable, and enjoyable, without being too restrictive and without cutting out any major food groups and without cutting out all the fun.

THERE ARE THREE components to any food plan:

- What to eat
- How much to eat
- When to eat

Most plans tell you what to eat but often skimp on instructions about how much to eat and when to eat it. In fact, many of us have been trained to believe that there are good foods and bad foods, aka foods that make us fat and foods that don't. This is false. There are no bad foods. There are no foods that on their own make you fat. However, any food can cause us to gain weight if we eat too much of it. (And any food can easily be overeaten if we haven't eaten in a while! But we will get into all that later.) First let's start with what is the most important part of any solid food plan.

WHEN TO EAT

I have found that the most important piece to the weight loss puzzle is when we eat. By eating early, we get our metabolism going and lose more weight throughout the day. By eating often, we keep our metabolism humming along and ensure that we don't get too hungry, which can lead to overeating. And by finishing most of our heavier eating early, we have most of our food intake finished before our metabolism naturally slows down for the day, at which point our food is more likely to sit—and store—rather than burn off.

Public Service Announcement (PSA): Your body's internal rhythms are aligned with nature, not with your bedtime. Even if you are up until 2:00 a.m., your metabolism slows down at nightfall. Finishing most of our eating early also provides the opportunity to incorporate the benefits of intermittent fasting, as I will explain later in this chapter.

How does this look practically?

Breakfast should be within an hour or two of waking up. Morning snack should be eaten no later than three hours after breakfast, and preferably even less. Lunch should be by 2:00 p.m. or earlier, and afternoon snack no more than three hours after lunch. Dinner should ideally be done by 7:00 p.m.

So, a typical day for someone waking up at 7:00 a.m. should look like this:

Breakfast: 8:00 a.m.
Snack: 10:30 a.m.
Lunch: 1:00 p.m.
Snack: 3:30 p.m.
Dinner 6:00 p.m.

Another variation, for those who have a bit of a later start to their day, would look like this:

Breakfast: 9:00 a.m.
Snack: 11:30 a.m.
Lunch: 2:00 p.m.
Snack: 4:30 p.m.
Dinner: 7:00 p.m.

Of course, there will be days that lunch or dinner may run a bit late, but let that be the exception to the rule—plan for success, not failure. This way you will be maximizing your metabolism and will never be too far away from your next meal or snack.

Also, don't be afraid to eat earlier if you find yourself particularly hungry. Many people have a fear of "running out of food" and going hungry when they are trying to lose weight. They "save" food for later, but in the meantime, while trying to prevent being hungry later, they are getting awfully hungry now. This becomes particularly true when you begin to eat early and begin to eat at regular two- to three-hour intervals, thus revving the metabolism. In other words, hunger is a good sign. If you find yourself hungry before the planned two-to three-hour mark, just eat. Here's what a sample day looks like for someone who is very hungry.

Breakfast: 8:00 a.m.
Snack: 10:00 a.m.
Lunch: 12:00 p.m.
Snack: 2:00 p.m.
Fruit: 4:00 p.m.
Dinner: 6:00 p.m.
Treat or fruit, if needed: 9:00 p.m.

See how I added the fruit in at 4:00 p.m., and voilà—no long gaps and no dramatic hunger.

Some of you may be wondering about intermittent fasting, as it is super popular right now. Intermittent fasting is a way of reaping the benefits of putting your body into a state of ketosis, which has proven weight loss and health benefits. It is my belief that it is sustainable for many people, when practiced moderately. You will notice that all of the schedules above integrate a fourteen-hour fast (with the exception of the third version, which incorporates a fruit or treat if needed). Fourteen hours is just enough time to achieve the benefits of ketosis.

Because eating early and eating often are essential to a maximized metabolism, I encourage people to only practice intermittent fasting if it is not at the expense of getting breakfast within two hours of waking up. Conversely, starting with breakfast at noon and ending at 10 p.m. would be a poorly planned fourteen-hour fast. Starting early, eating often, and ending early is the ideal way to get the benefits of ketosis without losing the benefits of the boosted metabolism. But if you need the option of having something a little later in the evening in a planned and controlled fashion, in my experience it is worth leaving that option open. Feeling too restricted can backfire.

BRAIN DRAIN

The most important key to weight loss is finding the right foods that promote weight loss and avoiding certain foods that make me gain weight.

BRAIN RETRAIN

The timing of my meals and snacks is potentially more important than my actual food choices.

6

SO NOW...HOW MUCH SHOULD I EAT?

I KNOW, I KNOW, you are all anxiously awaiting instructions for what to eat in order to lose weight. But I'm going to string you along a little more because, like I said before, it's not really about what you eat as much as when you eat and how much you eat. Of course, what you eat is important, but it's only part of the full picture. Let's keep going, in order of importance.

How much to eat in order to lose weight depends on various factors, including gender, age, weight, the amount of weight you want to lose, genetic predisposition, overall metabolism, and many other factors. Without knowing you, it is difficult for me to tell you how much to eat. Any book that offers a one-size-fits-all weight loss plan should stay on the shelves where it belongs.

I'm going to give you a handy rule of thumb that works for many people, but not all, and you may need to adjust this number if you find that it's not working for you. However, it is a decent starting point for many. It's a bit technical, so take this slow. Grab a calculator—I'll wait.

> **Step One:** Take your current weight and multiply it by 10.
> *Example*: 180 pounds x 10 = 1,800
> **Step Two:** Subtract about 15 to 20 percent from that number.
> *Example*: 1,800 x 0.15 = 270, and 1,800 – 270 = 1,530
> 1800 x 0.20 = 360, and 1,800 – 360 = 1,440

Someone who weighs 180 pounds should eat between 1,440 and 1,530 calories a day to lose weight. I would set her target at 1,500 calories a day in order to lose weight at a pace of about one pound per week.

Keep in mind that this is a very quick but rough formula that I have found to work, in order to set your target. It may need to be adjusted if you are losing too quickly or too slowly. But, like I said, time is on your side. Try it for a week.

Here's another example, this time for someone who weighs 200 pounds:

200 x 10 = 2,000
2,000 x 0.15 = 300
2,000 x 0.20 = 400
2,000 – 300 = 1,700
2,000 – 400 = 1,600

The target for this woman would be 1,600 to 1,700 calories a day in order to lose about a pound a week.

Here's one more, for someone who weighs 140 pounds (and likely doesn't need to lose very much, depending on her age, height, and other factors).

140 x 10 = 1,400
1,400 x 0.15 = 210
1,400 x 0.20 = 280

In this case I would recommend using the 15 percent target so as not to end up eating too little and getting too hungry.

So, 1,400 – 210 = 1,190, or approximately 1,200 calories per day in order to lose a pound a week on average.

These numbers may seem off because we are generally taught to eat a 2000-calorie diet, but in practice, this formula actually works. Also, bear in mind that I am erring on the side of caution because we tend to underestimate the calories that are in our food. We also tend to forget to count some calories, such as those in fruits, vegetables, and fats. Additionally, many food manufacturers adjust the calorie count on their nutrition panels by as much as 10 percent per serving, so I have factored that in as well.

I have found the following to be a good way to break up these calories:

Breakfast: 20 percent
Snack: 10 percent
Lunch: 20 percent
Snack: 10 percent
Dinner: 25 to 30 percent (approximately)
Fruits or treats: 10 to 15 percent (approximately)
Example A: A 180-pound woman would need to eat 1,800 calories in order to maintain her weight. Her target daily calorie intake for weight loss should be about 1,500 calories per day.

Breakfast: 20 percent = 300 calories
Snack: 10 percent = 150 calories
Lunch: 20 percent = 300 calories
Snack: 10 percent = 150 calories
Dinner: 25 to 30 percent = 400 calories
Fruits and Treats: 10 to 15 percent = 200 calories
Total: 1,500 calories
Example B: Sara weighs 220 pounds. Her target daily calorie intake for weight loss should be about 1,800 calories per day using the formula above.

Breakfast: 350 calories
Snack: 200 calories
Lunch: 350 calories
Snack: 200 calories
Dinner: 500 calories
Fruits and Treats: 200 calories
Total: 1,800 calories

If you prefer to have a larger breakfast or lunch, please feel free to adjust accordingly. It is actually better for your weight loss to have your larger meal earlier in the day, but I write it this way because, for many of my clients, this is the most practical.

THE GOLDILOCKS TECHNIQUE

While portioning our breakfast, lunch, and snacks can be as simple as glancing at the nutrition label and doing a quick calorie calculation, many people find it more challenging to determine their dinner calorie count. I have developed a powerful tool to easily figure out how much to eat that doesn't require any complex math or a calculator. I call it "The Goldilocks Technique." Here goes: Take a moment to picture how much dinner would be "too little," leaving you feeling hungry and susceptible to noshing around the house later at night. Now, picture how much dinner would be "too much," meaning you know you won't lose weight if you take that amount. Now, picture how much dinner is "just right"—that's the amount you should take. And now for the most important part. Take that amount and don't go back for more! Add plenty of vegetables so that you stay satisfied and stick to your decision!

This tool works well not just for dinner, but for determining how much challah, how much of a treat, and for many other situations where calorie counting is challenging. It is important to note, however, that if we haven't been on plan all day, or have gone for many hours without eating, this won't work well, as our hunger will have built up to the point where our judgment will be off. But in the context of having been on schedule, this is magic.

Ultimately, determining the exact amount to eat might take a bit of trial and error. Use the above as a starting point, and track your food portions while timing religiously for a week or two, and see if you lose weight. If you lose more than four pounds in two weeks, you may want to add some calories, as losing too fast can leave you physically depleted and set you up for failure later on. If you lose fewer than two pounds in two weeks, you may want to adjust your calories downward slightly so that you don't get frustrated by the pace.

A word of caution: These formulas are not exact science; they are a starting point for many people. Take the time to find your sweet spot, even if it takes an extra week or two.

BRAIN DRAIN

The most important key to weight loss is finding the right foods that promote weight loss and avoiding certain foods that make me gain weight.

BRAIN RETRAIN

When attempting to lose weight, portion control is potentially a more significant factor than my actual food choices.

7

AND NOW... WHAT TO EAT?

I KNOW, I KNOW, I am not being very helpful by writing a bunch of guidelines and leaving you to figure out what to eat on your own. You want me to tell you exactly what to eat, how much, and when. And I have mixed feelings about this because I feel I am doing you a disservice by telling you what to eat. You know yourself way better than I know you. And if I do tell you exactly what to eat, then here I am getting sucked into the trap of offering you a diet. Which I promised in the introduction that I wouldn't do. Goodness. Here is the deal: I am going to write a suggested plan for you that you can (1) follow exactly, (2) ignore completely, or (3) modify and customize as you see fit.

Ready? Okay, here goes:

Actually, please hold. Before we discuss what to eat, we would be remiss if we didn't discuss what to drink, and how much. What to drink, of course, is water. And the amount that you should be drinking follows a very simple formula: Take your weight and divide it in two. That's how many ounces of water you should be drinking per day. If you weigh 180 pounds, you should be drinking 90 ounces of water per day.

If you are dehydrated, your metabolism is about 10 percent slower than if you are fully hydrated. To clarify, this means that if you would normally burn 1,500 calories per day, you are only burning off 1,350. In other words, making sure you are fully hydrated gives you the equivalent calorie burn of taking a forty-minute walk. Without actually taking that walk. (And feel free to actually take that walk as well.)

Also, it is extremely common to mistake the feeling of thirst for hunger, so you'll be saving a couple hundred extra calories by not "thirst eating."

And here's a pro tip that I discovered over time—the same way we often don't feel hungry until we eat, we often don't feel thirsty until we drink. If you rarely feel thirsty, it might be because you are dehydrated. And if you want to feel thirsty, you might just need to get those first few cups of water in as early as possible, and that will activate your thirst mechanism (if that's a thing). And once it's activated, the rest of your daily water intake will be easier to manage, because you will be thirsty.

Okay, so now that I have sold you on drinking your water, we are finally up to the fun part: what to eat. What I am going to say now is shockingly simple. In fact, you may be disappointed, because we are so used to hearing all sorts of magical secrets to weight loss success. Okay, here it is:

- Whole grains
- Filling lean proteins (avoid too much saturated fat)
- Lots of vegetables and some fruit
- Healthy fats

Wait, that's it? Yup. Each meal should contain the above. Snacks should be delicious, satisfying, and have some sort of nutritional value. And don't forget to allow for some treats on a daily basis.

Let's create a sample day together using the calorie breakdown for our 180-pound woman mentioned above:

MEAL	WHAT TO EAT	CALORIE COUNT (APPROXIMATE)
Breakfast	Two slices of whole wheat bread + 2 eggs + lots of greens	300 calories
Snack	KIND bar	150 calories
Lunch	1 oz. of whole wheat crackers with 5 oz. of salmon + salad with 1 tbsp. of light dressing	350 calories
Snack	1 oz. of whole wheat pretzels + 1 tsp. peanut butter	150 calories

MEAL	WHAT TO EAT	CALORIE COUNT (APPROXIMATE)
Dinner	1 sweet potato + 5 oz. grilled chicken + a bowl of vegetable soup	400 calories
Add-ons	1 fruit + 1 Yasso bar or similar low-calorie ice cream	150 calories
Note: use add-ons where needed—either in the evening or between meals and snacks	Note: of course, feel free to swap out your starches, proteins, fats, snacks, and treats for the ones you prefer!	1,500 calories total

Okay, there we go. I did what I promised not to do. I wrote out a food plan. But really and truly, this book is not meant to be a diet. It is meant to be a way of life. This means that if you need to have a larger breakfast or prefer a smaller dinner, adjust accordingly. If you don't like the options I wrote, swap them for ones that you do. If you are going out to eat and aren't sure what the calorie count is, try to estimate and stick to clean proteins and vegetables. If you miss a meal or a snack, catch up as soon as you can—but don't delay the next meal or snack; just eat more closely together. Play around with different spices, seasonings, and cooking methods to keep things interesting. This is your show. This is your life. This is your food plan, so make sure that you love it.

BRAIN DRAIN

I need a complicated food plan created by a nutritionist in order to lose weight.

BRAIN RETRAIN

I need to make healthy choices so that I am full and sustained and set for success.

8
FAQS

HERE ARE SOME frequently asked questions about this meal plan:

Q. Are you sure this is going to work? It seems like way more food than I am eating right now.

A. Most of my clients tend to eat too little during the day and, therefore, have the impression that they eat quite little. However, comes 4:00 p.m. and they start snacking, munching, tasting dinner, eating the kids' leftovers, etc. They are actually consuming many more calories than they believe that they are.

They are in a lose-lose situation, where they are hungry all day and everything they eat sticks, because they are eating their food late in the day when their metabolism is slower.

More hunger + no weight loss = lose-lose.

By eating early and eating often, we maximize our metabolism and get to eat more food. Yay. This is why I put so much focus on the timing and the portion sizes. And yes—to answer your question that I can feel coming—if you eat all the food above but eat it later than the recommended schedule, you may not lose either. Stick to the schedule and the portion sizes, and watch the magic unfold.

Q. I weigh much more than the person above and need to eat more calories according to the formula you provided. What should I add?

A. You can add a few more ounces of protein, additional fruits, and/or higher calorie snacks. You can even add more carbohydrates, but don't go crazy.

Q. I weigh less than the person above and need to eat fewer calories. How should I adjust my food plan? Should I skip something?

A. I recommend that you reduce the calories *within* the meals and snacks by taking fewer ounces of protein and choosing leaner protein options. You can also leave off the carbohydrates by dinner, but don't leave them off for breakfast or lunch. Skipping meals or snacks and going long stretches without food isn't recommended because it slows the metabolism and doesn't allow you to lose weight as effectively.

Q. Why shouldn't I skip breakfast or lunch carbs? I don't feel like I need them.

A. You need to eat these, preemptively, so that you don't get too hungry later. Our metabolism is stronger during the day than at night, so the carbohydrates will burn off faster when eaten by breakfast or lunch. If you skip them and then get too hungry at night, you will likely need more carbohydrates by dinner, or find yourself hunting around the cabinet at night, which ultimately means eating more calories instead of fewer, at a time that your metabolism is at its lowest.

Q. I hate counting calories—is there an easier way to do this?

A. Yes. Estimate by using The Goldilocks Technique described above. This means that for each of your three meals you eat one plate of food. The plate is divided into three parts. Half the plate is filled with vegetables. A quarter of the plate is filled with healthy carbohydrates. And a quarter of the plate is filled with protein. Don't forget your two snacks in between meals. Do this for one week, tracking your food on a food log carefully as you go. (More on keeping a food log later.) Weigh yourself after the week is up. If you lose weight, keep going. If you don't lose weight, adjust your plate slightly by having less carbs by dinner, leaner proteins, lighter snacks, etc. Then repeat the process of tracking everything on your food log and weighing yourself at the end of the week.

Note: It is important to make sure that you aren't bloated when you weigh yourself.

Q. What do you mean by making sure that I'm not bloated?

A. There are certain foods that cause us to retain water, which can mask any weight loss that might have occurred. These foods include very salty foods such as feta cheese, lox, soy sauce, deli meats, and some vegetables, such as cabbage and eggplant. Avoid those foods twenty-four hours before you weigh yourself.

Q. I overdid it with one of my meals (or snacks). Should I skip my next meal?

A. No. This sets you up for a vicious cycle of overeating and under-eating, and then getting too hungry and overeating again. In this cycle, overeating usually emerges victorious. Rather eat a lighter meal such as a slice of bread with an egg white omelet or a yogurt and a few crackers.

Q. I know I have a big party later—should I skip a snack or a meal in order to save calories for the party?

A. Definitely not. Think about it this way. You are planning to eat at the party either way. The only question is if you are going to eat responsibly and moderately or eat with abandon. Coming to a party or a restaurant hungry immediately sets you up for failure. Skipping a couple hundred calories will end up leading to overeating by many, many more calories.

Q. I have a wedding (or bar mitzvah, or work event) at night, so dinner is going to be very late. I know it's important to eat dinner by 7:00 p.m.—what should I do?

A. Eat a few ounces of protein and some vegetables at around 6:30 p.m. before you leave the house. Then try to stick to proteins and vegetables at dinner.

Q. But then I'm eating double!

A. If you come starving you will end up eating triple. Also, notice we are avoiding carbohydrates because of the late hour, which should balance out the few ounces of extra protein. And guess what—you might not lose weight that day, but at least you won't gain. Not every day is a weight loss day. Some days are what I like to call "practice being a skilled dieter day." And not every night is an event—you will have your chance to lose weight, fear not.

Q. Why are fruits so limited? Aren't they healthy?

A. Fruits are healthy carbohydrates. They should be filed away in your mind in the same drawer where a slice of whole wheat bread is filed. Therefore, they have a place in the plan, but they are not unlimited. As far as their being healthy, this is true, but healthy food can also make us gain weight. Too much food of any sort gets stored as fat.

Q. Is there anything I shouldn't eat?

A. Again, there is no particular food that in and of itself makes a person gain weight. It's about quantity. That being said, avoid foods that aren't filling and can leave you hungry, as you may end up eating more. You should also avoid foods that trigger you. Meaning, if you know that once you get started with cereal and milk, you launch into a cycle of a little more cereal a little more milk until either the box of cereal or carton of milk is empty, avoid cereal and milk. If you know that once you start eating nuts or granola, or dried fruits, you can't stop, please avoid those, too. You are the boss. You know your triggers. If a food triggers you and leaves you hungrier after eating it than before you ate it, be smart. Stay away.

9

TRACK YOUR FOOD

ACCORDING TO SPARKPEOPLE.COM, a website that tracks the weight loss habits of millions of users, keeping a food log is the number one habit reported by people who lost more than thirty pounds and kept it off for more than five years. That means that if you make just one commitment, tracking your food should be it. Tracking every bite (you bite it, you write it!) allows you to remain aware and present at all times and keeps you accountable to yourself—it will keep you honest.

Often, my clients tell me, "I know what I eat—why do I have to write it?" This may be true, but it's a temporary state; meaning, most people, when beginning a new food plan, are hyperaware of every bite that goes in their mouth. Remember those honeymoon days, when everything in your day revolves around your new food plan, what you are "allowed" to eat and "not allowed" to eat? It's almost like there's a shadow around you, watching you, making sure you don't step out of line. We all have experienced this, but it is short-lived. Ultimately, our old habits creep back: we start trimming the edges of the cake just to even it out, we take a slightly larger portion of pasta, and we go back to bottom-feeding the kids' leftovers. So, even if you are aware of what you currently eat, take out a pen, and track your food. Make a habit of it.

Another claim that I often get is this: "I tried tracking my food, but it didn't help—I messed up anyway." To that I say, let's be reasonable. Tracking our food isn't going to cure us. If it was the magic cure, I would be out of a job and I would go take up Olympic swimming. It can't eliminate the "battle of the bulge," but if it helps us remain aware and accountable, that alone is a huge step. Take it. It literally takes two minutes a day. Think of it like flossing—easy, underrated, powerful.

Just this past weekend, my husband brought home glazed cinnamon buns from the bakery, *l'kavod Shabbos*. They come in a rectangle pan, a dozen glazed buns all stuck together. All Shabbos long I nibbled at the top of the buns, until Sunday morning, to my horror, I realized that the entire pan was still there, but with no glazed tops. Frantically I ran around asking everyone if they had eaten any of the bun topping. "No, Mom—only you do that thing where you destroy the food by picking off the best part. We haven't touched it." Grudgingly, I logged, "the top of twelve cinnamon buns" in my food journal. Had I not been in the habit of logging my food, each bite would have been insignificant, and I would never have realized how much I had actually eaten.

So, you see, I definitely understand the resistance to writing down our missteps. It makes it all too real. But that, indeed, is the point. Before we see it on paper, we tend to blur it out. Tracking keeps us aware and keeps us honest.

Of course, the main reason we don't love tracking our food is because it can be uncomfortable to look at our reality in the eye—we prefer not to know. To this, I will tell you, lose the judgment, and *lose the guilt*. There is nothing wrong with getting it wrong. It's simply a way to gather information and troubleshoot it, if desired, so that you do things differently the next time. I tell my clients that they should pretend they are reporting on someone else's food intake, as we tend to be much less inclined to report accurately about ourselves, often rounding down to the nearest reasonable portion (ever have the experience where you eat an entire sleeve of Oreo cookies and then write down "cookies" on your food log? Yeah, that's what I'm talking about).

I believe that the difficulty tracking our food religiously and accurately comes from shame, as if, somehow, we failed, and as if, somehow, this reflects upon our worth as a human being. I always tell my clients to try to think of their weight loss project as something a bit less loaded. Say you came to me trying to work on getting more sleep every night. And say you report back that you got to bed past 2:00 a.m. each night despite a firm commitment to turn the lights out by midnight. Would writing this "failure" down be as difficult? Probably not. It would be pretty easy to be fully honest and face it because it doesn't feel like a personal failure.

Somehow, though, dieting is different. I suppose it's because the food we eat actually ends up as part of our body; it suddenly feels like a moral failure. This is a sad reflection of the pressures and values of our society, but, with a little bit of rewiring, the shame and self-judgment can be overcome, which will, in turn, allow you to track your food more comfortably and with more accuracy.

Sometimes, I advise my clients to write down their food like a reporter or court stenographer—impersonal, impartial, simply collecting data. Gathering this information without judgment feels less personal but will still help you stay aware and accountable. It will help you focus your intentions for the week, help you troubleshoot ongoing areas of struggle, and even show you how much extra food you can "get away with" while still reaching reasonable weight loss goals.

I will advise against using any fancy apps for food tracking. By the time you are done searching the database to find the exact food (or, more often than not, finding a less exact match that reports the fewest calories), you probably need a nap. This isn't sustainable. Just grab a notebook and a pen and write down what you ate, what time you ate, and how much. Start a new page each day. Or use the notes app on your phone. Keep it simple so you don't quit. That's the motto here, you'll notice. In general, the easier and smaller the changes you make are, the more sustainable they are and the more likely you are to stick to it. Keep it simple.

BRAIN DRAIN

Tracking my food isn't helping. I know what I eat.
Or:
Tracking my food isn't helping. I am cheating anyway.

BRAIN RETRAIN

There's no reason for me not to take a good hard look at all the food I ate this week. It's not a moral or personal failure any more than not getting to bed on time, and will help inform the coming week. Self-reflection is key to growth.

10
ACCOUNTABILITY

DINA, A CLIENT I hadn't seen in over ten months, walked into my office. Dina had lost over fifty pounds, but I noticed right away that she had definitely gained it back. "Dina, I haven't seen you in forever! How have you been?"

"Not great," she answered. "I actually kept the weight off for several months. Then I got COVID-19 and lost about ten pounds in two weeks. When I recovered, I gained the weight back, and more. I thought I could lose the extra weight on my own, but week after week, I just kept gaining weight. Finally, my husband suggested that I come back to you because he saw how miserable I was. So, here I am."

I welcomed Dina back warmly, and asked curiously, "What took you so long to come back? If you saw you were struggling, why wait?"

"Honestly? I didn't want to be dependent on you. I wanted to show myself I could do it alone."

"Hear me out," I told her. "About 70 percent of Americans are overweight or obese. And the other 30 percent aren't immune from this struggle—most of them are struggling to maintain a healthy body weight. This means that there's nothing wrong with needing a bit of extra support or accountability—literally everyone does! Some get the help they need, and some don't, but almost all need it!"

I believe this perspective is important. We all want to be naturally thin and beautiful and don't want to be dependent on anyone or anything in order to be able to stick to our commitments. I get that. But what if we just accept our reality? What if we say, "I care a lot about this, but somehow, I just can't seem to do it alone, despite really wanting to." We need to ask ourselves, "Does not showing up for weekly accountability appointments mean I don't need anyone's help, or does it mean I'm just not getting the help I need?" You know from past experiences that this is not something you can do for a few weeks or months or even years and then just stop. For most people, if not everyone, we have to be committed to this for life. And that means finding a winning formula that not only gets the weight off but keeps it off.

In other words, reality check—you might have to have some level of accountability for a while, but in the grand scheme of things, spending a modest amount of time and money to manage one of life's biggest challenges is actually a bargain.

The irony is that most people understand the need for accountability during the weight loss process, but once they reach their goal weight, or close to it, they feel like they are done. This goes to the heart of the issue—if you go on a diet in order to lose weight, and then subsequently go off the diet, what do you expect to happen? For most of us, maintenance isn't a natural state of being. Our natural state of being is the state that we have been in most of our adult lives, which is the state of wanting to eat more food than we need. That doesn't change when we hit our goal weight.

Weight loss is only the beginning of this journey and is often the easy part. For many of us, the real challenge lies in developing the habits needed to keep the weight off. Whatever thoughts, habits, behaviors, and genetic makeup got us to our original overweight state, will ultimately get us back there—unless we continue with the new behaviors that we adopted when losing the weight: behaviors such as built-in accountability and support. If you found weekly accountability to be helpful to your weight loss process, follow through with some form of accountability, long after the weight is off.

BRAIN DRAIN

I can't depend on a nutritionist or food counselor forever—I need to do this alone.

BRAIN RETRAIN

I really do need the support. Denying myself that level of accountability doesn't mean that I don't need it. It's just denial.

11

A MUFFIN IS TWO DOUGHNUTS AND OTHER SHOCKING DISCOVERIES

THERE IS A COMMON misconception amongst dieters that if a food is healthy, it is weight loss friendly. This is far from the truth. The fact is that there aren't any specific foods that make us fat. It is too much food. Yes, that's right. Too much of most foods will make us fat.

I have a very health-conscious client named Mark with whom I have been working for some time. He is actually a cardiologist and sticks to a plant-based diet. After a few weeks of successfully shedding pounds, Mark's weight loss stalled and then stopped. I asked him to email me his food log so that I could troubleshoot.

Upon review, I noticed a lot of extra nuts and fruits on his food plan—a cup of Brazil nuts here, and a handful of dried mango there. When I asked him about it he self-righteously responded, "Well, that's my version of candy and chocolate. At least it's healthy!"

I gently pointed out to Mark that while healthy, these choices are very high in calories. And when we consume more calories than the body can use, the extra fuel will be stored as fat, regardless of how healthy it is. Indeed, his version of chocolate and candy is being utilized by his body as just that—chocolate and candy—extra calories being stored as fat.

In fact, sometimes healthier options can be even more insidious than unhealthy ones, as these foods allow us to drop our guard. While many of us wouldn't eat a doughnut from Dunkin' Donuts while on a diet, we may opt for a blueberry muffin because it seems like the better choice.

But believe it or not, the muffin can have twice as many calories as the doughnut.

Clients often ask me if it's possible that they are overdosing on fruit. While my inclination is to say no, when I press further, they tell me how they had an entire bowl of watermelon in one sitting—the equivalent of ten to twelve fruits, and the calorie and carb count of four packs of Skittles. So, yes, the fruit can indeed be the problem.

Many of us wouldn't touch chocolate cake but would likely have some carrot cake. And we wouldn't munch on chips at night but might feel more virtuous noshing on nuts. And while most of us would stay far away from a regular bagel, we may choose the whole wheat bagel and feel like we made a great choice, despite both bagels being very similar in carb and calorie count. (PSA: A large whole wheat bagel is equivalent in carbs and calories to six slices of bread.)

At this point you may be wondering why you should bother with healthy choices to begin with! Why not just focus completely on calorie count? Well, for one thing, healthy food is healthy. Oh right—*that*. But, secondly, nutritious foods are filled with fiber and protein that keep us fuller, keep our blood sugar steady, and make it easier to stay on plan. Eating a one-hundred-calorie chocolate chip cookie doesn't give us the same nourishment as a yogurt and a handful of blueberries. So, while technically one can lose weight by focusing solely on calories, it's mighty difficult to stay within a reasonable calorie count when you are malnourished and in a sugar coma. And that's leaving health out of the picture. So armed with this knowledge, be careful not to confuse health with weight loss. They are related, but kind of like second cousins.

BRAIN DRAIN

It's healthy, so it can't be bad for my waistline.

BRAIN RETRAIN

Too much food will get stored as extra fat regardless of its nutritional value.

12

TOO GOOD TO BE TRUE

THERE IS a very pessimistic saying that goes, "If it sounds too good to be true it probably is." We learn this when we are young, and we tend to believe it, especially as we get more cynical with age. But somehow, when it comes to dieting, we find a way to delude ourselves that there is a shake or a pill or a certain food that will be the answer, the elixir, the pill, the cure to our weight loss woes. Allow me to act as your convenient little naysaying voice of reason. There isn't. It won't.

Unless you confront yourself and face your thought patterns, behavior patterns, and habits, and do the hard work of pushing through, you will always hit the same dieting wall.

This little adage is true about nutrition labels as well. If the light brown, vaguely whole-grain-looking, deliciously squishy four-ounce pita claims to be whole grain and one hundred calories, think again. Manufacturers are not above fudging the numbers. Even hedge fund managers and accountants, with a lot more to lose, fudge the numbers. If the numbers on a nutrition label seem off, they probably are.

I can't tell you how many clients texted me asking me if Tic Tacs can count as "free," meaning to ask if they can be eaten freely without fear of consequential weight gain. Indeed, the packaging claims that Tic Tacs contain zero calories. But the answer is, "No, ma'am." Tic Tacs aren't free. They have approximately two calories per Tic Tac, which doesn't seem like much until you find that you ate the entire two-hundred-piece container, netting you a cool four hundred calories—definitely not free.

And you might be interested to know that even manufacturers that aren't intentionally misleading you can be rounding down the calorie count by as much as 10 percent. The FDA legally allows a 10 percent margin of error, and manufacturers use this as a way to make their products appear to be lower in calories than they actually are. This is so common that it is almost standard practice, which causes problems for those of us following a food plan that involves calorie counting.

The reason I tell you all this is because if you have been on your food plan for some time, and your weight loss has stalled, you might want to double-check to make sure there aren't any "too good to be true" foods that are sabotaging your progress.

You may be wondering, "I have been eating the same foods all along, and I didn't have a problem until now—even if the foods are higher in calories than I originally thought, they can't be the source of my stalled weight loss, can they?" The answer is very simple. As you lose weight, your body needs less fuel to sustain itself. What may have started out as a weight loss plan could ultimately stall and turn into a maintenance plan. The way out of this plateau would be to cut some calories. But before cutting anything from your base plan, do a quick scan to see if there are any "too good to be trues" that need to now be eliminated. There's often a fine line between losing weight and maintaining your weight, and, sometimes, these little things are the tipping point.

BRAIN DRAIN

If the label states a certain number of calories, it must be true even though it seems off.

BRAIN RETRAIN

If a nutrition label doesn't make sense to me, it's likely inaccurate, either because it's intentionally misleading or because of manufacturing loopholes. I'll cut that food out for a week and see if it helps me get back to losing weight.

13

THE GREAT SCALE DEBATE

SHOULD I WEIGH MYSELF every day? Once a week? After each bite? Never? There are good arguments to be made for most of the above options.

Let's start with the school of thought that tells you to weigh yourself every day.

Pros: The good part about daily weigh-ins is that knowing that we are getting on the scale the next morning tends to keep us in check and serves as a bit of accountability throughout the day.

Cons: Weight loss isn't linear. Any food plan that has you losing more than two pounds a week is likely too drastic and, therefore, bound to backfire, which means that you won't be seeing much of a difference from one day to the next. For many people, this could be frustrating and discouraging.

There are so many factors at play, including hormonal fluctuations, constipation, bloatedness, erratic schedules, etc., which can all temporarily affect your weight.

As you may have experienced, the daily weigh-ins can take on a life of their own. I have clients who report stepping on and off the scale ten or fifteen times a day, and I am sure some of them are underreporting. When we go on the scale too often, we are usually hoping for some sort of alternate reality. Either I overate and now I'm hopping on the scale to see if I somehow miraculously got away with it, or I have been disciplined about my food plan, and I'm feeling so pleased with myself that I'm hoping I lost four pounds since the last time I stepped on the scale six minutes ago.

Getting on the scale tends to elicit intense emotional reactions. Our day can be ruined by an unsatisfactory number on the scale. Husbands can be yelled at, kids can be snapped at, and coworkers suddenly become extra annoying if we are not pleased with the scale's readout. And how many of us have stepped on the scale after a few days of hard work, and, if the number wasn't to our liking, felt ready to quit our food plan, even though we had been feeling fabulous right until we decided to step on the scale. And then, suddenly, we feel fat. So, no need for a constant readout.

Then there are people who don't weigh themselves at all. They just go by how they feel or how their clothes fit.

Pros: You save money on a scale. And batteries aren't needed in this scenario either. You also free up time to do things other than weighing yourself.

Theoretically this may be ideal because the main objective of any weight loss program is to feel great and under control, both of which can be accomplished without ever seeing a number.

Cons: Practically, this tends to backfire. Whenever we set goals for ourselves, they need to be SMART. SMART means Specific, Measurable, Attainable, Realistic, and Time-based. In order to track progress and change course, if necessary, there needs to be some sort of measurable progress. Feeling great is hard to measure, and clothes fitting, while somewhat more measurable, is also kind of vague. Hello, elastic! So, getting on the scale on some sort of regular basis is an efficient way to measure progress.

Of course, the scale should never be the only measure of success—not at all. In fact, I make sure to ask my clients how they are doing before they step on the scale. I find out how they feel about their week, their progress, their level of consistency, their struggles, and their victories before weighing them. Often, they'll answer, "Well, let's see what the scale says," and I tell them, "No way! The scale is secondary—the main thing is you!"

In general, I recommend that my clients weigh themselves weekly, preferably on a consistent day and time. We don't want to track their weight minute by minute like a heart rate monitor, but we do want a consistent measure of progress.

BRAIN DRAIN

Every time I feel like I worked really hard, or, alternatively, every time I feel like I overate, I go to the scale for feedback.

BRAIN RETRAIN

I know how I'm doing based on how I'm doing. I don't need the scale's constant opinion. Once a week will do.

14

DON'T HOPE—MAKE IT HAPPEN

> **ME:** "Bye, have a great week, and make sure to stick to your food plan. See you next week!"
>
> **CLIENT:** "Thanks, I hope I'll do great."
>
> **ME:** "Wait one second—come back for a minute. If you are leaving my office hoping for a great week, we still have work to do!"

Dieting isn't about hoping. Hope implies that it's out of your hands—that it's really not up to you. Of course, no one is completely in control of their life, and things happen all the time, but hope just seems so vague and fatalistic. You need to know your plan of action.

Do you have a master shopping list? Do you have a menu for the week? Are you preparing lunches to take with you to work? Is your fridge stocked with fresh fruits and vegetables? Do you know where you want to keep your food log? Do you have a water bottle? Do you have reminders set for things you often forget about? Is there cake on your counter or chocolate in your cabinet waiting patiently to be removed? Are there schedule changes that need to be considered? There are so many factors that are under your control that hope hardly seems necessary. Make some moves. Take action. Take control.

I often find that my clients are able to stick to their plan right up until something happens that's out of the usual routine: a snow day, a busy day filled with many errands, a wedding, a birthday party, etc., and suddenly the food plan goes out the window. But, unless there is some sort of emergency, almost all these things can and should be anticipated and planned for. We can't just stay on plan when it's convenient—and we know more about what to expect in each of these situations than we care to admit. Even the non-routine days are relatively predictable. This Yom Tov season will likely look very similar to last Yom Tov season, and your next family vacation will probably pose very similar challenges to the last vacation. You can safely assume your kids will drive you crazy, and that you will need another vacation when you get home. And you can also anticipate your food challenges on vacation. If we take a moment to think about what's coming up, we can plan for it, and we won't have to rely on hope.

I call this Dieting Through. We tend to diet *around*: "I'll diet *after* the holiday or vacation or birthday celebration, but not during. This mentality often comes from a punitive view of dieting. Most weight loss diets seem to be asking, "What's the least you can eat without killing you? Great, let's have you do that!" Well, if you hate your diet, there's no way you are willing to Diet Through life's celebrations or tribulations. Life would just be depressing.

But as you may have noticed, my perspective on weight loss is slightly different. I like to ask, "What's the most enjoyment and pleasure that we can have from food without sacrificing our weight loss goals? Great, let's do that." With this mindset, we can Diet Through anything because we don't have to starve or cut out any major food groups or even eliminate fun in order to reach our weight loss goals. We just need to make a plan that we feel good about and then stick to it. And remember, we believe that not every week is a weight loss week. But every week is an opportunity to build skills and habits.

Different times call for different plans. The same way we may budget money differently on vacation from the way we do on a day-to-day basis, we might want to adjust our food plan as well. While the goal during routine, normal days may be to lose a pound a week, the goal during Pesach or Sukkos may be to shift focus toward sustaining our habits and maintaining our progress.

Say I'm going to Miami for a quick getaway. Many would say, "Alright, I'll diet when I get back; I just want to have fun while I'm there." The problem with this mindset is that a free Shabbos with no restraints is hardly fun. We tend to overdo it to the point of physical and emotional discomfort and walk away from each restaurant feeling regretful and bloated. When we have free reign, we tend to take it too far.

But what if we rewrote our rules before we even got to the airport? What if we took a few minutes to consider, "What does vacation mean to me? What do I need in order to make it feel fun and social?" Personally, this would mean having a steak at a nice restaurant without worrying about the portion size. It would also mean having at least one or two margaritas by the pool, and I'd probably need an ice cream at some point while strolling the boardwalk.

But that's pretty much it. Sure, I would also love French fries, fried chicken, endless alcohol, and all-you-can-eat buffets. All. The. Time. I would love it, but I would also regret it—and I don't *need* it in order to feel like I'm on vacation. And I can still eat the rest of my meals and snacks according to plan. I can still drink my ten cups of water, and I can still track my food intake. And best of all, I can come home from vacation with my suitcase and souvenirs, without being laden down with pounds of extra weight on my hips and the heavy burden of regret.

Eating eight ounces of extra steak, three margaritas, and an ice cream cone over the course of a week will not sabotage my diet. While I'm not likely to lose weight while I'm away, I am also unlikely to gain too much, and anything I do gain I will be okay with, knowing that I chose it, planned it, and stuck to my plan. By putting some structure into the unstructured, by making some rules for the exceptions to the rule, I can truly have the best of all worlds.

BRAIN DRAIN

I don't want to diet on vacation or at parties. I just want to have fun. I'll worry about it later.

BRAIN RETRAIN

Life is always busy, and there will always be a reason not to diet. I can stick to most of my food plan, most of the time. I will allow myself what I need in order to still enjoy myself without regrets later.

15

RUN YOUR DIET LIKE A BUSINESS

A COUPLE of years ago, I read a well-known self-help book titled *The 4-Hour Workweek*, by Tim Ferriss. While some of the suggestions in the book are already quite dated, the main message still holds up: work smarter, not harder. While this book was written to inspire people to free themselves from the nine-to-five grind, I found that many of the concepts work well for dieters. Yup, that's just where my brain goes—I can't help myself.

Dieting takes time and energy. In fact, I often find that the two main factors that determine whether or not a dieter will be successful are time management and emotional regulation. We'll discuss emotional regulation in upcoming chapters, but for now, let's take a look at our time management skills. Many of us lead busy lives and feel like we don't have enough time to eat right. The truth is that many of us do have some spare time; we just don't have spare time at the *right* time. Mornings are hurried, our daily tasks eat into our lunchtimes, and the pre-dinner rush is almost universal.

Well, if dieting takes time and energy, let's give it the time and energy it deserves. If we treat dieting like a job or a business, we can make sure we are dieting as efficiently as possible, that we are on top of our game rather than trying to do everything at once and scrambling to keep up. There is no need to reinvent the wheel every day. We can have systems in place to make sure things are running smoothly.

Ferriss uses the acronym DEAL, which stands for Definition, Elimination, Automation, and Liberation, as a handy way to keep things running efficiently. (I changed Definition to Delegation and tweaked this acronym a bit to suit our purposes.)

Delegation. The boss can't do it all—that's why he has employees. This is not a new concept, but in *The 4-Hour Workweek*, the author challenges the reader to be more aggressive about delegating, encouraging us to only do what can't be done by others, freeing ourselves up for what is most important or necessary. Let's apply this business concept to the business of dieting. Have your daughter, or even your cleaning help, prepare you a salad. Ask your husband to take over homework duty so you can focus on preparing a healthy dinner. Appoint someone to make you a smoothie in the morning. Have a friend call you each night to see how you are doing with your food plan. Ask the people around you to help you refrain from eating foods that you know you will regret later. Delegate any task that doesn't *have* to be done specifically by you.

Elimination. If you are running out for copy paper every time you run out, and then running out for ink three days later, you aren't being very efficient. For those of us who feel we don't have enough hours in our day, consolidating and thereby eliminating tasks can free up precious time. The same holds true when trying to run our diets efficiently. Eliminate unnecessary runs to the supermarket by making thorough lists. Buy prepared vegetables to eliminate preparation and clean up. Skip the coffee line by ordering ahead, freeing up time for more important things like preparing lunch.

Automation. Just like we have our bills on autopay and our thermostats preset, try to figure out which parts of your food plan can be automated. Can you have a set weekly shopping list? Can you set alarms to remind you to track your food or drink your water? Whenever possible, set it and forget it, so you can worry your pretty little head about other things.

Did you ever notice that you can either check your text messages or emails one hundred times a day or twice a day and be similarly productive both ways? Checking one hundred times a day is inefficient and distracting, while checking and responding twice a day gets similar results in a fraction of the time. Apply this to your food plan. Rather than preparing chicken cutlets for grilling several times a week, buy a family pack and prepare a month's worth while you are running a production line anyway. Rather than cutting a salad for the next day's lunch, prepare three days' worth and store it in the fridge. The more you work toward automation the more efficient you will be.

Liberation. Now that your day is running smoothly and automatically, you have liberated your day. You have freed up critical time when you need it most, and now, this time is yours. Use it to schedule all the healthy eating habits that you couldn't find time for earlier.

BRAIN DRAIN

I don't have time to eat right.

BRAIN RETRAIN

I have time for anything that's important to me. I can utilize effective time management strategies to make the time. I just have to want to do it.

PART II

WHEN THE **GOING** GETS TOUGH

INTRODUCTION TO PART TWO

THIS SEGMENT of the book was written with the understanding that we don't always eat because we are hungry. We are triggered by many different things, and understanding our emotional triggers can help us be more prepared to deal with them.

Common triggers include the following:

- Life worry/stress
- Stress about weight
- Feeling like a failure about your food
- Feeling like a failure regarding other areas of life
- Feeling overwhelmed
- Physical pain
- Fatigue
- Boredom or understimulation
- Feeling judged, rejected, or blamed
- Intense emotions, either positive or negative
- Hormonal fluctuations
- Interpersonal conflict
- Distorted thinking patterns
- Desire to rebel or assert control
- Restricted eating that we bring upon ourselves
- Restricted eating imposed by others
- Anxiety or tension
- Need for pleasure
- Deficit of coping skills or emotional regulation

In the coming chapters, we will learn how to handle ourselves when the going gets tough and develop the thought patterns and habits that we need in order to successfully stick to our food plans.

While I mostly approach this section logically, I also believe that many of the challenges listed above can be tackled on a spiritual plane as well. It is my belief that much of our emotional angst has spiritual roots. When we are connected to Hashem and understand that our purpose in life is not simply to have comfort or pleasure, but to grow, our struggles and discomforts take on new meaning.

When we are worried, stressed, or feeling insecure, turning to Hashem and relying on Him is not just a helpful tool—it is literally the point of our existence. Hashem has perfectly designed us, our circumstances, and the entire world. Conducting ourselves with the knowledge that every moment is uniquely designed for our benefit is the most powerful self-regulatory tool. Of course, knowing this in our heads and feeling it in our hearts are not the same thing. Making a daily spiritual practice of connecting to Hashem, or *hisbodedus*, is key to being able to access this level of knowledge when it is needed the most.

16

WHEN THE HONEYMOON IS OVER

ALMOST EVERYONE STARTS their diet off strong. We float on a cloud of weight-loss-induced bliss, perfectly following every single part of the plan, reading the instructions over and over like it's a Bible. But at some point or another, the thrill wears off, temptation gets the better of us, and, sooner or later, our old habits come creeping back in—not usually all at once, but rather bit by bit, until there's nothing left of the original plan.

When this starts happening, my clients often complain to me, "I don't know what happened! I used to be so strong and so motivated, but I seem to have lost my self-control!" To which I respond with the sobering truth: "You never really had it. The initial thrill and excitement of your new food plan was fueled by adrenaline, not self-discipline. When this wears off, you are reintroduced to your regular self with all the same habits, desires, and struggles that you always had."

I like to compare this to the honeymoon phase of new relationships. When a couple first gets together, there is usually a period of bliss. Communication is easy, flaws are overlooked, and every quirk seems endearing and adorable. But eventually, the newness wears off, and ultimately, the couple has their first fight. And just like that, the honeymoon is over.

Now, the couple may wonder what happened—they used to have the most amazing relationship. But the truth is that their bliss wasn't due to them being excellent communicators and amazing partners—it was a temporary adrenaline-fueled override of their natural selves. At this point, some couples split up and date other people in an attempt to get back that high. Others push through. They learn to deal with their differences, work through some of their issues and hangups, communicate, and, ultimately, reconnect—often on a deeper and more meaningful level than before.

When my clients feel the initial stage of inspiration has worn off, I ask them to view it as a milestone. And an inevitable one at that. I help them see this new stage for what it is—an opportunity to take a good hard look at their habits, beliefs, and struggles surrounding food and begin to tackle them in a real way. While the honeymoon phase feels good and gives the weight loss process a head start, the real work has now begun.

Like our squabbling honeymooners, some dieters will go find a shiny new diet. They aren't ready for the real work and prefer to feed off the newness—the high. But those who tough it out end up dealing with their weight loss struggles in a deeper, more profound, and more lasting way. My advice—stick to your plan and work through your issues. Use this next stage to face the old thought patterns and their subsequent behaviors, and replace them with shiny brand-new ones that are more conducive to your long-term goals. No diet (or relationship) can keep you high forever. Embrace the opportunity to get to know your real self. The honeymoon may be over, but say hello to the satisfying long-term relationship.

BRAIN DRAIN

I don't know where my self-control went. I used to be so strong!

BRAIN RETRAIN

Now that the adrenaline rush is over, I am excited to start rethinking about my habits so that I can stay the course.

17

DO WE EVEN HAVE INTUITION? DO WE NEED IT?

INTUITIVE EATING is all the rage. Tune in to what your body needs, eat when you are hungry, stop when you are full, and all will be well with the world. Like many other dieting concepts, I believe in this in theory. However, we need to at least consider the possibility that our intuition might be a little bit broken.

If you had a coffee and your kids' leftovers for breakfast, skipped lunch, and had a diet coke and a protein bar somewhere in the middle of the day, and now want to listen to your intuition, you're pretty much doomed. You won't be able to determine what you need or distinguish hunger from cravings, because you are undernourished and sugar spiked. You will likely feel very justified in eating everything in sight, because you *feel* like you hardly ate. Your intuition is not likely to help you make good choices or practice portion control. Your intuition is gone, and survival mode has kicked in.

Similarly, if you spent the past hour watching baking reels on TikTok and now you're roaming around the kitchen trying to figure out what to eat, you may be tempted to make something that entails pounds of dough, sticks of butter, and globs of cheese—once again, your intuition has been influenced by outside forces and is hardly trustworthy.

And if you're at a party surrounded by tables laden with sweets and pastries, and you're three or four cocktails in, and everyone around you is eating like it's her last day on Earth, your intuition will fail you, yet again.

So, how do you practice intuitive eating? The first step is to establish a solid baseline. Once you are on a predetermined food plan that includes scheduled meals and snacks, moderate portion sizes, and nourishing food choices from all the food groups—eating in a structured, regulated way for some time, and your blood sugar and appetite are stable—you can start tuning into, and trusting, your intuition.

I have a client who came to me after years of diet hopping. She had a complicated relationship with food as well as a binge eating disorder, and was desperate to stop the cycle of starvation diets followed by binge episodes. We created a plan that she felt was suited for her, and she followed it carefully for several weeks, tweaking it whenever she felt it was needed. She was very successful at first, and finally felt that her binging was under control, mostly due to not being deprived.

Then, one week, Sara called me for our scheduled phone sessions, and told me she had binged on some sugar-free chocolate bars she had bought for her husband, a diabetic. I asked her what triggered the binge, and after thinking about it, she figured it out. She had been reading an article about intuitive eating over Shabbos, and it struck a chord with her. She decided (on the spot) that she had always felt that she needed more fats in her plan, and decided that chocolate was the answer.

This is what I mean by our intuition being broken—adding fats in the context of a discussion would have been listening to her intuition. Eating those chocolate bars because she read a book on intuitive eating served to justify a craving. I reassured Sara that we do believe in intuitive eating, and reminded her about all the different changes we had made to her food plan along the way. But using our intuition needs to be done cautiously, as cravings and temptation can easily masquerade as intuition.

The main thing to be cautious about is not to rewrite the rules on the spot, as you go. For example, if you know that when you are expecting your period you always crave chocolate, you might want to officially add two ounces of chocolate to your food plan without guilt when that craving arrives. Having a strategic baseline and then making adjustments based on the patterns we notice will allow for more consistent weight loss than classic intuitive eating alone.

This pragmatic approach allows us to recognize our behavior patterns and be prepared for them in a proactive manner. This allows us to be less dependent on our often-fickle intuition.

BRAIN DRAIN

I am going to just practice intuitive eating. I like the idea of eating when I am hungry and stopping when I am full.

BRAIN RETRAIN

Intuition is a fickle friend. Objective structures and boundaries, as well as proactive planning, will allow me to differentiate intuition from cravings and temptation.

18

INTUITIVE EATING (CONTINUED)

WHEN TO TRUST YOUR INTUITION

IF YOU HAVEN'T noticed by now, I have mixed feelings about intuitive eating. I find that intuition is a fickle animal, that can be blocked, swayed, and influenced quite easily. Therefore, the belief that if we eat when we are hungry and stop when we are full will result in our maintaining a healthy body weight is theoretically ideal but challenging in its practical application.

Here are some examples of ways our hunger can mislead us:

- It's very possible that I may get very busy and not notice my hunger even if it's present, the same way I don't always run to the bathroom the moment I feel the urge.
- It takes about twenty minutes for the hunger mechanism to activate, and, I don't know about you, but twenty minutes is plenty of time to eat and overeat. If I get busy and skip a meal, I will likely be too hungry to eat intuitively, or I may eat too much too quickly, before my fullness radar kicks in.
- If I eat something loaded with refined carbs, I will experience a spike in blood sugar, followed by a crash. I will immediately feel hungry even though I have already had plenty of calories.
- Certain situations or settings can activate a Pavlovian response, where we feel hungry even if we just ate. For example, walking past the bakery aisle in the supermarket, watching a cooking reel on Instagram, walking into my mom's kitchen, etc. These situations trigger the urge to eat, hungry or not.

The list goes on and on, but the message is clear: our desire to eat can't always be trusted. So, when can we trust it?

If you are sticking to the guidelines in chapters 5–7, you can trust your hunger. Meaning, if you are choosing healthy and filling foods, eating every two to three hours, and generally sticking to your plan, and then you suddenly notice that are feeling particularly hungry, trust that hunger.

There are many reasons why you may feel hungrier than usual that are actual legitimate reasons, not based on faulty intuition. For example, for a woman, the days leading up to her period—with its hormonal fluctuations—can leave her a bit hungrier. Another example: you may have had a more active day than usual. Even mental exercise such as poring over a complicated spreadsheet can leave you feeling a bit hungrier than usual.

In order to make sure that you are actually hungry, I recommend that you do a quick two-part self-checkup:

- Is the hunger coming from my stomach, or do I feel it in other parts of my body? If it's not coming from my stomach, it's not hunger.
- Do I want a specific food, or will anything do? If I want something specific, it is more likely a craving, and not really hunger. When we are hungry, we will pretty much eat anything.

If you determine that the hunger is real hunger, you had best eat something. The main reasons that most traditional diets fail is either because we are feeling too hungry, or we are feeling too deprived. While most of us can tolerate hunger in the short term, I don't recommend fighting legitimate hunger. Our bodies are designed to maintain homeostasis and will probably overcompensate for the perceived deprivation when the opportunity eventually presents itself.

What you eat and how much you eat is up to you. Keep in mind that when your brain signals that you are hungry, that doesn't necessarily indicate an emergency. Because you have been eating regularly every two to three hours, the hunger signal is regulated to the point that it's more of an indication light than an emergency light. Hunger means *eat*, but doesn't mean *panic overeat*.

Have some fruit, yogurt, or a slice of whole wheat bread with some peanut butter on it, and see how you feel after twenty minutes. Don't worry if it's more than you originally planned to eat or more than the food plan that you created allows. Your body needs it—respect your body. If you still don't feel better after twenty minutes, eat your next scheduled meal or snack. Don't worry about "using up your food" or being hungry later. You are hungry now. Eat now. Later will likely sort itself out.

BRAIN DRAIN

I am afraid to eat more than planned because it might make me gain weight.

BRAIN RETRAIN

If I am eating nutritious food at regular intervals and have performed a quick body scan, I can trust my hunger, and trust that it's what my body needs, without fear of gaining weight.

19

YOU ARE NOT THE VOICE INSIDE YOUR HEAD

WHEN MY CLIENTS go off their food plan, I ask them to tell me what they were thinking before they dove into chips. Often, their first response is, "I wasn't thinking—I just ate." I maintain that this isn't so. Eating isn't like breathing—it's not automatic. Whenever we eat something that isn't on our food plan, we are aware of it, at least momentarily. During this split second, we actually need to quickly justify our upcoming action, in order to reconcile it in our brains. This can happen so quickly that we may not even realize it, but it's definitely happening.

When pushed, clients will tell me all sorts of original justifications. Okay, let's call them what they are: excuses.

Here are some of the most common ones:

- A little bit won't hurt.
- It's healthy, so it's okay.
- I skipped lunch, so this is instead of lunch.
- I'll fix it tomorrow by eating less or working out more.
- I deserve it.
- I'm too stressed to worry about it right now—I just don't care right now.
- I can't be perfect all the time—it's not even good to be too perfect because I'll get my body used to that.
- Balance is important.
- Everyone around me is eating much more.
- I already lost enough weight this week, so I'm allowed.
- I already messed up, so I might as well keep going.

Does any of this sound familiar? No, I am not psychic, and I'm not reading your mind. I'm reading mine. And the list goes on and on, becoming increasingly creative as needed, because, basically, the brain is like a little child having a tantrum who will say or do anything to get his or her way. In the span of a few minutes, it can tell you, "You already lost enough weight this week—you're a winner; go for it!" And five minutes and seven Oreos later, it'll tell you, "There you go again—you messed it all up. Don't even bother trying anymore. Just give up and keep eating." Wow. You went from a winner to a loser in the span of five minutes. Impressive work there.

What in the world is going on here?

Hang tight—I'll explain. Hashem created this world in a way that we have complete *bechirah*, free will. This means that whenever we want to do something positive, there will always be a negative counter-effect creating resistance. Otherwise, it would be too easy to do good, and therefore, there would be no value in our good. The reward and the growth require resistance. This being the case, as soon as we decide we want to take charge of our health, a decision that would ultimately be good for us and benefit us, we are bound to be met with resistance.

This resistance can be thought of as an echo—we have a thought to choose to prepare a salad rather than eat a slice of kokosh cake, and then our brain starts to echo with voices of doubt.

"I'll just have a bite."

"I deserve to relax."

"I already lost weight this week, so I can afford it."

"I just have to taste it so I don't insult my mother-in-law."

Etc., etc., etc.—you know the drill. Our brain keeps churning until we come up with something valid enough to allow us to buy in, because that is the way the world was created. And it echoes so loudly that we begin to believe that it is actually our own voice; we identify with these thoughts because it is more comfortable to remain stagnant than it is to grow. Once we buy in, we are then free to eat what we had our eye on, pretty much guilt free—of course, until the guilt sets in. We can remain in our comfort zone without guilt.

And it all happens so quickly we may not even realize that we are identifying with the echo instead of with our true self. How do we stop ourselves from going down this road? Well, you have already accomplished the first step. The first step is to hear the echo, recognize it, and embrace it. It means you are on the right track, because there will always be resistance to anything positive.

Metacognition—being aware of your thoughts, particularly those that allow you to go off plan—is super useful for helping you resist them. We are creatures of habit, and even our thought patterns are habitual. The unhelpful thought that sealed the deal for me this time has probably gotten me one hundred times before. But once we are aware of this thought and behavior loop, we can change the pattern, and change the habits. Often, just being aware that the voice of resistance is supposed to be there and that it is part of the growth process is enough for many people, but for more helpful tools, refer to the next chapter.

BRAIN DRAIN

I am having all these unhelpful thoughts, and they actually sound true. I'm sold. I'll give in this time and then get back on track later.

BRAIN RETRAIN

All positive actions will trigger a negative counteraction, because change and growth require resistance. I don't have to listen to or identify with the echoes.

20

DO NOT NEGOTIATE WITH TERRORISTS, YOUNG CHILDREN, OR THE VOICE INSIDE YOUR HEAD

AS WE SAID BEFORE, the problem with these habitual unhelpful thoughts (HUTs) is that they always have an element of truth. Your brain would never say, "Well, the chocolate is brown, and all brown foods have zero calories, so dig in." Nope—that would insult your intelligence. But it may say something like, "Well, it's sugar free. And I read that fats are good for me." And I may find myself deeply involved in a family-sized bar of chocolate before I can reconsider.

Once you are aware of your HUTs, what's next? The first rule of thumb is this: Do not engage in a back-and-forth argument with these thoughts. You will always lose. The addict inside will come back at you with an argument that is even better, stronger, and more compelling.

Think of it like a child whining for a candy bar in a grocery store.

> **CHILD:** "Please, Mom, please can I have that candy bar?"
>
> **MOTHER:** "No, honey, it's going to spoil your appetite for dinner."
>
> **CHILD:** "But I promise I won't eat it until after dinner."
>
> **MOTHER:** "Yes, but if I buy you one, all your brothers are going to want one also."
>
> **CHILD:** "Well, I promise I'll only eat it in my room, so they can't see."

MOTHER: "I know, sweetie, but it's not good for you."

CHILD: "Well, I'll eat only fruit at snack time in school for the next two days. Please, Mom, please!"

We all know how this conversation ends.

As you see, by engaging with your child, you are actually getting closer and closer to giving in with every explanation you give her. Our HUTs are the same way—the more you engage with them, the closer you are actually moving toward giving in.

What can you do? Simply put, acknowledge the HUT, thank your brain gently for bringing it to your attention, but stand firm in saying no. If saying no feels harsh, you can say, "Not right now," or "Not today."

Back to the whining daughter, imagine if the conversation went like this:

CHILD: "Mom, can I please have a candy bar?"

MOM: "No, honey, I'm sorry."

CHILD: "But I promise I'll eat dinner nicely."

MOM: "No, sweetheart, I said no, and I meant no. Maybe another time."

CHILD: "You are so mean; you never let me have anything."

MOM: "I know you feel that way, and I understand how disappointed you are, but I said no, and I'm sticking to it."

While standing firmly by the original no without engaging in a logical back and forth will likely result in a sulky child, it will also result in a child who knows that her mom means what she says. And next time she hears no, she'll likely accept it sooner and with much less nagging.

Step one is to be aware of the HUTs that justify our going off plan. Step two is to disengage from the battle inside your head by firmly telling the unhelpful thoughts no. That's it. Just no.

Remember, our brains can only handle one thought at a time, which means we are in full control of each and every thought. Our thoughts are quite cooperative and willing to go in new directions. The more we practice this skill, the more natural it becomes. This is how new thought patterns are formed, and our behaviors and habits follow!

BRAIN DRAIN

"A little bit won't hurt," "I'll fix it tomorrow," or any other potentially true but particularly unhelpful thoughts along these lines.

BRAIN RETRAIN

Aha! I recognize that thought process, and this time, I'm not going down that rabbit hole. While this thought might have some truth, it isn't a helpful thought, and I have the power to change my thoughts to more helpful ones, leading to more helpful behaviors.

21

IT'S NOT YOU, IT'S THE FOOD

SOMETIMES YOU MAY be unsure if you're hearing the echoes of resistance that come with progress, or if you have a legitimate concern that would interfere with your ability to stay on track. Here's a good way to break it down for yourself, but bear in mind that if you have the presence of mind to evaluate the legitimacy of certain thoughts, you are already a step ahead, and more likely to make decisions that you feel good about in both the short and long term.

Think back to the habitual unhelpful thoughts (HUTs) discussed in the previous chapter. They all have truth. They are all logical. And I'm sure you can come up with even more compelling logic.

- I don't want to insult the host or hostess.
- I need to taste this to make sure it came out good.
- I can't throw away food or waste it, so I need to eat it.
- I'm not going to have a chance to eat this again, so I had better take advantage.
- My weight loss shouldn't be so important to me; I should have less vain goals.
- It's dangerous for me to diet if I'm pregnant or nursing.
- I don't want to give my children an eating disorder by being strict about my food.
- I can't keep away from this forever, so I might as well give in now.
- I'm a cranky mother when I feel deprived, so I'm eating this for the sake of my family.
- It's unhealthy and even bad for my weight loss if I'm too stressed, so I need to do some serious stress eating right now.

While none of these are inherently false, and, in fact, many of these unhelpful thoughts have solid elements of truth, we need to question if the logic truly holds up.

Here's the logic litmus test. If there is no food dangling at the other end of this logical argument, it may have some validity. But if the logic appears in the presence of food, it is now subject to questioning, because we have lost all objectivity. We aren't thinking. We are feeling an urge, and we justify it with our thinking.

The best way to handle this questionable logic is to validate that there may be some truth to these arguments, but to recognize that you are in no place to make logical decisions, as your judgment is currently skewed. Not only that, but when you made your commitment to stick to the plan, your judgment was clear—in other words, you were of much sounder mind when you made your commitment than you are right now, feeling the urge of cravings, hunger, stress, emotional hunger, etc.

If you determine that your logic is indeed being influenced by the promise of food, tell yourself you will think about it for a little bit before deciding. Tell yourself that you will discuss it with your nutritionist or weight loss buddy and get right back to yourself shortly.

BRAIN DRAIN

I have really compelling reasons for giving in this time and eating this cheesecake. This time it's for real.

BRAIN RETRAIN

As a general rule of thumb, I can't trust my logic when there is food at the other end of this "logic."

22

NOW YOU HAVE THREE SECONDS...3...2...1...GO!

NOW, FOR SOME good news. Just like we have unhelpful thoughts that gently lead us off plan, we also have empowering thoughts, which we will call Habitual Helpful Thoughts (HHTs), that help us stay on plan. Think about the last time you resisted something that you really wanted. What was your thought process that helped you resist? When I ask clients this question, I usually hear some variation of the following responses:

- I didn't want to mess up my weigh-in tomorrow.
- I thought about how I would feel after eating it.
- I thought about my upcoming wedding, vacation etc., where I want to look my best.
- I told myself that I can't get into the habit of always giving in; I need to learn to resist and strengthen my self-control.
- I know I won't be able to stop at a little, so I figured it's not worth starting at all.

These HHTs are often much less deeply rooted in our brains, simply because we give in much more often than we resist. Therefore, these thoughts don't come quite as readily as the unhelpful thoughts. But guess what—they could. You just need to resist more often rather than give in. The same way our HUTs appear to us so easily, the HHTs can become second nature as well.

The difficulty with the HHTs is that because they are little baby sapling thoughts, they can easily be overpowered a moment later when the HUTs come back rearing their persistent, ugly heads. And in the spirit of full disclosure: your brain will become increasingly more creative with the HUTs—if the old thoughts no longer get you eating chips and chocolate, your brain will come up with newer, more compelling HUTs.

Having said that, once you have identified your most common HUTs and learned to respond to them and shut them down gently and firmly, it is time to learn to replace those HUTs with HHTs. Stay with me here, we are going to do a little exercise. Quickly visualize a green balloon. A purple balloon. A purple grandmother. A green puppy walking a purple grandmother on a leash...you still with me? I'm sure you kept up—our thoughts are amazingly flexible and cooperative. Despite our deeply rooted habitual thought patterns, we can train our brain to have newer, more helpful thoughts, if we put our minds to it.

HUT: "I am going to count this milkshake as my fat for the day because I didn't have a fat for lunch."

HHT: "I have heard that one before, and I'm not falling for it this time. I am going to resist the milkshake now, and I'll get some frozen yogurt as a snack tomorrow. I prefer to exercise my self-control, and I am excited to fit into that dress that I just bought."

Boom! No back and forth. No falling for the old thought patterns. And creating new and empowering thought patterns and habits all in one split second.

There is one last step to this exercise in order to ensure successful resistance. The final step is to follow up your "power thought" with an immediate "power action." Perhaps you are about to dig into some leftover pizza. You have a fleeting thought about your upcoming trip to Cancun, where you are planning to wear a new bathing suit. You have a moment of inspiration; this is when you must act. Throw the pizza in the trash. Or walk away from it. Or make an announcement to whoever will listen that you aren't eating any pizza.

Mel Robbin's book *The 5 Second Rule* posits that we have about five seconds from when our power thoughts hit until the inspiration wears off and the unhelpful thoughts creep in, which means you have about three seconds to act. Get used to acting fast. Spit it out, throw it in the trash, give it away, remove yourself from the scene—do whatever it takes to see this power-HHT through. Because, while it may seem like a small battle, we need to win as many as possible as often as possible, in order for these thoughts to take root and become second nature. As the saying goes, "It doesn't get easier; we just get stronger."

David Hamelech was onto this way before Mel Robbins was. He writes in *Tehillim*: "*Sur mei'ra va'aseh tov*—Turn away from evil and do good."[1] We tend to think of this as two separate things—turn away from evil, and also do good things. I would like to posit that he may have meant that in order to conquer something that is challenging for us, we must not only turn away from it, but immediately do good—immediately make a power move by doing a positive action; otherwise we might end up right where we started.

BRAIN DRAIN

Once I find my helpful thoughts, the battle is over, and I can let my guard down.

BRAIN RETRAIN

Finding my helpful thoughts is empowering, but for the battle to be over, I have to take quick, decisive action!

---

1 34:15.

23

BE A MAN (OR WOMAN) OF YOUR WORD

WHAT IF I CAN'T ACT? Maybe it's not practical to run out of the room or spit out my food. Good news—you're not out of options. As long as you can speak, you are good to go.

Think about something you want to get done today. Now, write it down. Now, say it out loud. Do you feel the difference between thinking it, writing it, and saying it out loud? We have a million thoughts per day, so when we think about something it doesn't necessarily mean it's going to happen. If every single thing we thought about actually came to fruition, we would be completely overwhelmed and would never get anything done. Our brain doesn't really take our thoughts too seriously. One way to filter which thoughts warrant action is to write them down. This is why we make shopping lists, menus, and work calendars. But an even more powerful tool, and one that is highly underutilized, is simply saying things out loud.

Our words have value. For most of us, we don't say something unless we really mean it. Let's harness this for our own good. Picture the following scene: It's Thursday night, which means pizza night in my house. Usually, I have one slice of pizza and a diet coke on pizza night. However, on this particular Thursday, I had already eaten a large lunch, and really didn't want to eat any pizza. Thinking to myself that I really don't want to eat any pizza isn't going to be very effective once the cheesy, lightly browned, bubbling hot dish is set in front of me. Writing down my alternative dinner plan—an omelet and some grilled vegetables, may be somewhat more effective. But imagine if I gathered my five children and announced, "Guys, I'm going to pick up the pizza, but I am just letting you know that I don't want any and don't plan on having any. I'm having an omelet instead."

Well, now I'm bound by my words. I am far less likely to eat the pizza than if I had just left it as a free-floating thought, like all my other free-floating thoughts that come and go throughout the day.

And to make this even simpler, when announcing your intentions, you don't necessarily need to have anyone around. Try it and you'll see. Saying it out loud, even to the walls, solidifies your commitment and holds you somewhat accountable—because our words are worth something.

BRAIN DRAIN

I want to stay on track, but it's not always practical to act on my positive thoughts the moment that I have them.

BRAIN RETRAIN

My words have power. I will say my intentions out loud and drown out the noise in my head.

24

YOU ARE WHO YOU EAT (WITH)

IN THE FIRST SECTION of this book, we discussed dieting efficiently as a time management tool. One of the suggestions was to delegate, and I mentioned getting family members involved. I believe this to be important enough to warrant its own chapter, as the people with whom we interact on a daily basis can have a profound effect on the way we eat.

I grew up in Chicago as one of nine children, five of whom were boys. I was sandwiched between two of those boys, one being a year older than me and one a year younger. Once a week, we had pizza night, and my mom would usually order at least three 18-inch pies in order to feed the masses. It was always slightly competitive and stressful—my brothers would go hard at the pizza, taking their second slice before I was even halfway done with the first. I didn't even know if I needed a second slice, or a third, because that was hardly the point. I just grabbed myself another slice every time they did, in order to lock in my fair share.

Fast forward to about ten years later, when I first met my husband. We would stop at his favorite pizza joint, and he would ask me what I wanted. I would ask him what he was having and invariably he would say an olive slice. Trying to appear polite (I'm not, but at the time I still wanted to appear as if I was), I would tell him I'd have a slice as well. A slice. Singular. Turns out that without the stress and competitiveness created by my brothers, I was actually pretty satisfied with just one slice. That was when I first came to the realization that the people around us affect the way we eat.

We can take this positive peer pressure and use it to our advantage. If you have people in your home who are supportive of your weight loss journey, you can utilize this to your advantage, assuming that the help comes in a non-judgmental manner.

My family is under strict instructions not to allow me to eat junk food at night. I usually have a pretty easy time staying on track all day, but, like many of you, after dinner is when the real challenge begins. When we are all hanging out in the living room, I gravitate toward junk food like a moth to a flame. So, my teenagers, husband, and even my ten-year-old twins are all well trained to help me exert self-control.

However, this has to be done right. When someone asks, "Are you sure you want to be eating that?" The normal reaction is to feel judged and defensive. "Of course I want this. I'm eating it, aren't I?" But I have found that when taught to ask in a more helpful manner, the defensiveness is gone. My husband now asks, "Am I supposed to be stopping you?" This takes away all the judgment and allows me a moment to consider whether I really want to be eating what I'm eating. And oftentimes, my non-defensive response will be, "Yes! Please take this away from me!"

Even my children are on Mom Supervision Duty. My daughter is the keeper of the chocolate. When there is chocolate in the cabinet, I tend to not eat it responsibly. But I am not willing to subjugate myself to a life without chocolate. I have her in charge, and she hides it. When I want some chocolate, I ask her for it. She asks me how much I want, and I tell her. She then brings it to me, and even if I want more afterward, the answer is no. Once I am in my sugar bubble, I can no longer be trusted. I told her what I wanted when my mind was still clear, and I am bound by that—no changing my mind.

Realizing how the people around us affect our food choices both positively and negatively is an important piece of the weight loss puzzle. Give it some thought, and see if any changes need to be made.

BRAIN DRAIN

I have to have what everyone else around me is having. It's only fair.

BRAIN RETRAIN

The people around me can derail me or help me stay on plan. I am the master of my life, and the choice is mine.

25

NO, YOU DIDN'T BUY THAT FOR THE KIDS

WHEN DISCUSSING lifestyle changes, one of the most common refrains that I hear is, "I would be happy to shop and cook healthfully, but I can't deprive my family," or, "I host a lot, and I need to serve good food to my guests." I totally get it—if your family is used to having homemade cookies when they walk in the door after a long day, there may be an all-out uprising when you try to shake things up. And if you are famous for your homemade pies, you might feel uneasy about disappointing your guests.

But let's be honest with ourselves. Sometimes, it's not about the family or the company. How many times do we pick up a cheesecake from the supermarket and think to ourselves, "Mmmm...yummy! Caramel cheesecake! I'm having dinner guests this week—let me buy one of these for dessert."

If we would stop and analyze our thoughts for a moment, we would realize we have zero intention of not having it at all. We are definitely having some—we are buying it because we like it. We are probably telling ourselves that we will have enough self-control to eat it in moderation, but we are definitely having some of that cheesecake. And even if we have struggled to eat this particular item in moderation in the past, optimism seems to always prevail. If we are fully honest with ourselves, we will find that a lot of what we feel we have to do, we actually choose to do. In fact, the person who will have the hardest time with these changes might very well be ourselves.

Try to shop and bake with the mindset of *What's the most delicious food I can buy or make that my family will enjoy but that is still resistible to me?* If I'm a sucker for blondies, I'm better off baking brownies since I find those somehow easier to resist. If I can't resist cheesecake, maybe it's better for me to buy an ice cream cake when I'm having guests so that I'm not overly tempted. Don't think of this as selfish; we don't all have the same taste buds or the same triggers, so the others will very likely be happy with either choice. But this way, *you* will have a much easier time sticking to your plan.

Take a few minutes to take stock of the foods you buy or make for your loved ones, and ask yourself honestly if they need it or if it's really *you* who wants it. Doing this may challenge how you define yourself as a hostess or as a mother or wife. Be ready to feel a bit of loss or disappointment when you decide to let some foods go. Just remember, letting go of something before it's made or bought is infinitely easier than resisting it once it's already in front of you.

BRAIN DRAIN

I have to buy these cookies/candies/cakes for the kids.

BRAIN RETRAIN

Let's be honest: I can instead buy them things they will enjoy but that don't particularly speak to me.

26

SPEND SOME MONEY, HONEY

A 2017 STUDY of over three thousand women found that the first thing adult women worry about is their children. No shocker there. But take a guess what the number two worry was. If you guessed world events, reproductive health, the purpose of life, career or financial issues, health issues, aging, or any other highly concerning thing, you would be wrong. Our number two concern is our waistline.

Let me ask you this. If you had the following two choices—(1) you would be financially stable and never have to worry about money again, but you had to remain obese forever; or (2) you would be financially uncertain or even unstable, but you would remain thin forever and never have to worry about gaining weight again—which would you choose?

Many of us would choose the latter, as the study I referenced above confirms.

Of course, there are exceptions to every rule, so if this doesn't apply to you, or seems overly dramatic, don't shoot the messenger. Whether our waistlines should be our second-to-highest priority is a conversation for another time, but in the meantime, for many of us, this is the reality. The part that is even more illogical is that we are so concerned about our weight, but when it comes to investing our time and resources to facilitate change, we balk.

We hesitate to buy ready-cut vegetables or pre-seeded pomegranates because they're expensive, but we end up eating gummy bears instead. We schedule appointments and meetings through our lunch break even though we know we will pay the price later—coming home too hungry to think clearly and heading for a tub of ice cream sets the tone for an evening that spirals out of control.

To be fair, I believe we do this because we underestimate the importance of these small investments. We don't realize how much the precut vegetables or the deliciously prepared fruit will help us. And we minimize the effect of a skipped lunch, without considering how many times that same skipped lunch resulted in a sloppy, disorganized evening.

We tend to forget that once we slip, we often spiral. We tell ourselves, "I'll start again tomorrow." And then tomorrow comes, and we get on the scale and see that our weight is up because of last night's mess. We begin to feel that all our efforts are going nowhere, and we lose our motivation, all because of a handful of gummy bears or one skipped lunch.

If you are part of the 74 percent of women whose weight is one of their top two concerns, start acting like it. Invest your time and money wherever possible, even if it seems wasteful. The return on the investment will be worth it, I promise.

Here are some suggestions for people who are short on time but still want to prioritize their weight loss:

- Buy grab-and-go veggies, such as baby carrots, snap peas, mini peppers, and cherry tomatoes. None of these require too much prep, and they don't need immediate refrigeration.
- Subscribe to a meal delivery service. There are several kosher options in the tristate area. While some of them require subscribing to a full food plan and can be quite expensive, others will happily deliver á la carte—you can order lunch or even just dinner, straight to your door.
- Buy grab-and-go meals. A ready-made salad, a bought turkey wrap, a tuna sandwich on whole wheat bread, or even a container of chickpeas can serve as a decent lunch—it just means having the forethought to add these items to your regular shopping list. If you are concerned that there is too much fat in the mayonnaise or too many calories in the wrap, you can always leave over a portion of the food.

- Have your household help assist in meal prep. An hour or two per week should do the trick. It's less expensive than hiring a private chef, and much less expensive than paying someone to help you lose weight your whole life.

The key here is to stay in the solution rather than the problem. Instead of staying stuck in the "I don't have time to take care of myself" rut, try thinking creatively—remember, this is a top priority!

BRAIN DRAIN

I don't have time to prepare properly or the money to take shortcuts.

BRAIN RETRAIN

This is extremely high on my list of concerns and deserves an adequate investment of money and time, at least commensurate with the level of importance my weight loss is to me.

27

THE PERFECTIONIST AND THE OPTIMIST (PART 1)

SEEING CLIENTS in private and group settings day after day for over ten years has afforded me some insight into different dieter profiles. Two of my most struggling dieting types are (1) the Perfectionist and (2) the Eternal Optimist.

More on the Eternal Optimist in the next chapter—for now let's discuss the Perfectionist.

While perfectionism has its advantages and disadvantages, when it comes to effective dieting, perfectionism is usually more of a hindrance than a help. My perfectionists tend to see every deviation from the plan as a complete failure.

Perfectionists tell themselves that it's all or nothing, black and white, on my diet or off my diet. They are the ones who tell themselves, *I have already gone off track, so I might as well finish the bag of chips/the day/the Shabbos/the weekend*. If you are familiar with the thought process of "I anyway ________, so I might as well ________," you are likely engaging in the black-and-white thinking of a perfectionist.

Imagine if we applied this sort of thinking across the board. I popped one tire; I may as well pop all four. I tripped on the first step; I may as well just toss myself down the entire flight of stairs. I had one argument with my husband; I may as well go looking for a new spouse. The comic opportunities here are endless.

How do we fall into this illogical thought pattern that borders on insanity? Very simple. Dangling just past this faulty logic is...well, I don't know what, but it's likely something delicious. Something compelling enough to allow ourselves to temporarily fool ourselves into actually buying into this nonsense. Because unlike the popped tires and broken bones, this line of thinking ends up with...cheesecake...chocolate...freedom! I don't have to try anymore! I tried and I failed and now I am free! At least, until I am desperate again.

We need to learn to validate the frustration and disappointment of not having a perfect week without letting it derail us. This is a skill just like any other skill. A skill that can be learned with repetition, time, and practice, just like all the other thoughts, practices, and behaviors outlined in this book.

This isn't to say you should get sloppy on purpose. Do the best you can. But if you do mess up, embrace the opportunity to practice living in the gray—being less than 100 percent but forging on.

What if we redefine success and, therefore, failure? What if we told ourselves that good enough is good enough? What if, instead of the goal being to adhere perfectly to our food plan, we made it the goal to stick to our plan well enough to lose some weight each week? This completely changes our definition of failure and eliminates the black-and-white thinking.

While many diets ask you to eat as little as possible for as long as possible, how about telling yourself that you will eat as much as possible while still consistently losing weight? This type of calibrating doesn't mean you can do whatever you want whenever you want. You still need a basic food plan that will allow you a general amount of weight loss each week, and you still need to keep an excellent log of what you are actually eating, but you don't have to be perfect. You just have to be good enough. And while perfect may be fastest, good enough lasts longest.

You may want to find a new mantra to replace "I already messed up my perfect week; I might as well keep eating." You might say something like, "It's disappointing to fail, and I may not end up seeing weight loss this week, but at least I get the chance to practice being gray. I'm getting back on plan, now." Embrace the gray, as it's pretty much here to stay.

It is inconceivable to think that there is any way to be perfectly on plan forever. Get used to messing up and bouncing back.

My friends, if you grabbed a couple of potato chips—toss the rest of the bag in the trash, jot it down in your food log, take a glass of water and a deep breath, and continue on your merry way. You look great in gray!

BRAIN DRAIN

I already messed up, so I might as well just enjoy myself now, and I'll get back on plan after Shabbos, Yom Tov, vacation, etc.

BRAIN RETRAIN

I already messed up. But I can swallow my disappointment at my inability to get it 100 percent right and get back on plan, now. Perfectionism has no place in the growth process.

28

THE PERFECTIONIST AND THE OPTIMIST (PART 2)

HOW MANY TIMES have you been told that it's better to be a pessimist than an optimist? I'm guessing not too many. If you are hearing it now for the first time, I am honored to have the privilege of being the one to tell you. Let's discuss the benefits of optimism versus realism in the context of dieting, and see if you agree with me.

We all know that there are certain foods that tend to trigger us more than others. It may not even be our favorite food. For example, we may be able to resist the cake on the counter, but then will eat four handfuls of almonds, telling ourselves they're healthy. Or we may bring home pastries from a party, telling ourselves they're for our kids, but then end up eating them all before they wake up.

Sometimes, we see something we love in the supermarket and buy it, even though it's not on our food plan. We tell ourselves it's for our husband or children, but somewhere in the back of our honest minds, we know the truth. We know we will be eating at least some ourselves because, after all, we are buying it because *we* love it! How do we fall for it over and over again? The inner dialogue goes something like this: "I am going to buy this for my kids because I love it, and they will, too. But hopefully I won't eat it. But I really love it, so hopefully I'll just have a little bit." And before we know it, the item has made its way into our cart, into our homes, and, ultimately, onto our waistlines. There is the optimist, hard at work, convincing us that this time will be different, and this time we will somehow have more self-control.

When we buy or make foods that trigger us and that we tend to overeat all the time, telling ourselves optimistically that this time we will get it right, is simply fooling ourselves. In this situation, it's better to be a pessimist. Imagine if the inner battle went something like this: "Last time I bought a case of soft-baked chocolate chip cookies, I was also watching my weight, and last time I brought it into my home, it was also very well intended, and last time I also hoped to allow my family to enjoy it and hoped that somehow I would just take moderate portions, and how did that turn out? Not well! So, why would this time be any different? Let me put these cookies back on the shelf." Pessimism saves the day!

When discussing this with clients, I am often asked, "But why should my family suffer just because I am watching my weight—my children are all thin!" I usually laugh and tell them that, first, no one is suffering without soft-baked chocolate chip cookies the size of a frisbee. Those cookies are unhealthy for anyone, thin or not. Not bringing them home isn't "causing your children hardship."

Second, let's evaluate the inner logic to see if it holds up. The logic is that I'm going to buy my favorite chocolates because I don't want to deprive my children, and I will hope to eat them responsibly and resist the rest of them. Well, if it were that simple to resist, why not resist it right here and now in the grocery store? Let me guess—because it is irresistible.

Third, you are buying your favorites because *you* like them, and you are justifying this by saying your children need them. That makes no sense. I'm sure your kids would enjoy them, but they don't need the very item that triggers you. There are plenty of choices out there that you can buy when you legitimately want to treat the children that are less triggering. Buy them something that they enjoy, but not the very things that you find irresistible.

I recently ran into my local supermarket on a Friday afternoon to grab a few last-minute items for dinner. As I rushed past the bakery section, I noticed a rack of freshly baked sourdough challah rolls and loaves that looked like they were hot out of the oven. The sign read, "Buy any two items, get the third free." I loaded up, grabbing a bag of challah, a pack of rolls, and a loaf of sliced challah, filling my arms with the heavenly softness of the freshly baked deliciousness.

My inner voice was screaming with caution that this could be a dangerous purchase because fresh challah is my downfall, but I silenced it by saying that the kids would be excited about it, as sourdough challah recently became all the rage. I slipped very easily into the delusion that the sourdough bread was for the kids.

Hands full, I went on to grab the items I originally came for. As I adjusted the loaves in my arms to make space for a bottle of ketchup, I looked down at the nine pounds of challah that I was holding and almost laughed.

You see, a serving of sourdough bread is approximately one to two ounces of bread. "What are the chances," I asked myself, "that out of the 288 ounces of fresh challah in my hand, I would eat only two to four ounces over Shabbos?" Um...zero.

I know my fresh challah track record all too well. And thankfully, I had the presence of mind to ask myself the question that we should all learn to ask ourselves: "If I haven't been able to resist fresh challah in the past, and I can't resist buying it now, how do I expect to resist overeating later?" And so, resignedly, I put the challah back on the shelves, and went to the register to ring up my bottle of ketchup.

I am not going to lie—it wasn't easy. But it was worth it. And take a guess whether my children suffered. Of course not. They were never privy to my internal battle and never even knew that those pounds and pounds of sourdough challah almost made it into my kitchen and onto my waistline.

Being optimistic that, somehow, I would be strong enough to eat this fresh-from-the-oven deliciousness in perfect moderation would have actually been delusional. Learning from my past experiences and knowing my triggers has turned me into a successful pessimist. And the relief I felt when I left that store is hard to describe—you just need to experience the thrill of realism for yourself to know what I'm talking about.

BRAIN DRAIN

I love these ______ (fill in the blank)! I am going to buy them for my family, and hopefully, I will only have a little, if any.

BRAIN RETRAIN

I love these ______ a little too much, and whenever I buy them I tend to overdo it, despite my best intentions. I'm going to avoid this battle and just not buy it. Phew! Feels good to be honest with myself!

29

"STRESS EAT" LIKE A PROFESSIONAL

IN THE PREVIOUS CHAPTERS, we threw the phrase "stress eating" around. This can also be called "emotional eating." Emotional eating is any eating that takes place either intentionally or unintentionally, with the distinct purpose of relieving intense emotional discomfort.

While many professionals discourage stress eating, I believe stress eating gets a bad rap. I think of stress eating as functional and helpful, but you need to learn to do it like a pro. Hear me out. When clients come to me to discuss emotional eating, they generally come to me looking for tools or ideas or some sort of magic to stop their stress eating. I ask them to look at it differently. "First of all," I explain, "let's be clear. The problem is not the stress eating. The problem is whatever the stress-inducing problem is." Whether it's their marriage, their job, their children, their inner angst, or any number of problems that we adults contend with, the stress eating isn't the problem. If anything, it's part of the solution. At least a temporary solution.

However, for emotional eating to be a real part of the solution, it requires some skill. Think about emotional eating like taking Tylenol for a headache. The headache is the problem. Tylenol is the temporary solution. Taking two Tylenols will alleviate some of the problem, but taking twelve Tylenols will not provide six times as much pain relief. You may no longer have a headache after twelve Tylenols, but that will be because you are unconscious. We stop after two Tylenols, whether we got rid of the headache or not.

Circle back with me to emotional eating. If we can make sure to keep our stress eating moderate and controlled, it can actually serve as part of the solution. This means utilizing food as a de-stresser but not depending on it as our only emotional regulation tool in our toolkit.

Picture this scene: You come home exhausted after a rough day at the office. You are a little bit concerned about your son's reading disability. You are exhausted from your day, but there are still dishes in the sink that aren't going to wash themselves. Your chest feels a bit tight with worry, your back is tense, and you have a feeling in the pit of your stomach.

As you straighten up the counters and run through what you should have said to your boss if you were only strong enough to stand up for yourself, you notice a sleeve of Oreo cookies sitting on the counter, left there by your dyslexic but adorable eight-year-old. Just one cookie, you tell yourself. You deserve it. Plus, you went on the scale this morning and you were already a pound down, so you can get away with it.

You eat the cookie, and your shoulders start to relax as you are flooded with endorphins, not dissimilar to the effects of crack cocaine. Just one more, you tell yourself. Two cookies won't ruin a week's worth of work. And the pit in your stomach eases up a bit when you reach for the third cookie. You decide you'll do an extra ten minutes on the treadmill in the morning. By the fourth cookie, you tell yourself, "Forget this; I'll start my diet tomorrow."

Drumroll please. This is your green light to go ahead, no more questions asked, no more excuses needed; you are free to indulge until tomorrow, because tomorrow you will be really determined, and tomorrow you will be really committed. Seven or eight more cookies follow, and this ends one of two ways—either the Oreos are gone, or you suddenly notice that you once again aren't feeling too great.

What started out as an endorphin-releasing, muscle-relaxing drug that helped you temporarily forget your boss, your kid, and your dishes is now a stomachache combined with the familiar and distinctly uncomfortable feelings of regret, failure, guilt, and disappointment.

What went wrong? The first Oreo felt so lovely. It actually eased your stress and worries for a moment. The answer is that you took it too far. Once you ran out of plausible justifications (refer to Oreos 3 and 4 for reference), you gave yourself permission to not need to give yourself permission. Once you took the route of "I'll start again tomorrow," you effectively gave yourself permission to stop excusing yourself. And then all bets are off, and the only way out is when the discomfort of the food you are eating or the regret you are feeling outweighs the discomfort of the original problem. And now you are left with two problems. Oh boy.

Let's analyze this episode from a physiological perspective. Stress produces cortisol. Cortisol in moderation is a means of survival. Cortisol prepares the body to deal with stress or danger. In proper doses, cortisol helps control blood sugar and blood pressure. It also helps regulate how the body uses food and gets energy—your metabolism. For the most part, fight-or-flight—otherwise known as acute stress—is a good thing. If you suddenly see a car swerving into your lane and your body triggers a stress response, you will be able to respond quickly and maneuver out of the way. And even when the body responds this way to a non-threatening situation, like the need to perform well at work, or closing a deal, it can still be beneficial, because it gets you geared to perform at full capacity.

The problem is that, today, the fight-or-flight response is more likely to come from situations such as hosting the in-laws, figuring out what to wear to a party, or even just thinking about something that makes you anxious. Problems begin when acute stress is triggered by societal or mental stressors rather than physical stressors, as commonplace as paying your bills, sitting in traffic, or even responding to an email. Your body is prepared to act, but there's not much it can do to get away from the perceived threat.

In response to the perceived stress, the adrenals release greater and greater amounts of cortisol, ultimately resulting in adrenal fatigue. Adrenal fatigue is thought to occur when the adrenals have become overtaxed by excess cortisol release and can no longer produce levels of cortisol necessary for optimal body function.

Adrenal fatigue is linked with numerous mental and physical health issues, including the following:

- Anxiety
- Depression
- Digestive issues
- Headaches
- Heart problems
- Difficulty sleeping
- Weight gain
- Problems with memory and concentration

In other words, the prolonged high cortisol levels prompted by chronic stress are thought to cause these problems.

We must reduce our stress. That's a given. And if we are in a place where we are tuned in emotionally or connected spiritually, this would be a good time to utilize some of the skills and tools that we have developed. But, sometimes, we can't see past the food. If we are going to use food as a drug in order to temporarily self-medicate, let's do it. But let's do it right.

Here's the hack. Take the cookie. Take two. Bring your level-ten stress down to a level seven or eight. But after those two cookies, pause, revel in the pleasure of feeling a bit better, even temporarily, about whatever plagues you, and then move on to other stress management tools to continue lowering your stress level.

While food may be first, and food may be best, once our anxiety has been lowered to a level seven or eight, we are in a much better position to use some of the other emotional regulation tools that help relieve our stress, such as journaling, taking a hot shower, calling a funny friend, hitting a punching bag, or taking a few deep breaths.

BRAIN DRAIN

Right now I just don't care—I'm going into a food coma and will meet you on the other side. Bye!

BRAIN RETRAIN

I am staying present and in the moment. I may be self-medicating, but I can do this without overdosing. I will then be in a better position to effectively manage my stress in other ways.

30

THE MAKING OF A BINGE

IN MY PRACTICE, I find that there are two types of emotional eaters: Stress Eaters and Binge Eaters. There are different ways of thinking about both of these, but the general consensus among mental health professionals is that binge eating is a disorder, while stress eating is just a manifestation of poor stress management skills. I believe that it's a bit more complex than that.

Emotional eating and binge eating are similar, but binge eating is an even deeper-rooted survival mechanism. Binge eaters describe themselves as going into a trance and not remembering what they ate. They also say that they will literally eat anything—it doesn't even have to taste good—which is different from stress eating. This makes me think that there is something deeper and more primal going on. And, in fact, most binges are triggered by something in their day that actually activates a deeper trauma, usually from childhood.

When childhood trauma is triggered, a person's very survival is felt to be at risk, in a very real sense. The most recent studies surrounding trauma indicate that trauma develops when there is a threat, whether physical or emotional, during which the child feels helpless. Rather than fight-or-flight kicking in, the third option, freeze, is activated. Freeze is the terror of not being able to fight or flee, and not being able to help oneself survive. Don't make the mistake of thinking that there has to be an actual risk of immediate death. The body perceives danger to itself in many ways—abandonment, embarrassment, and feelings of inadequacy can all be perceived as imminent danger to the body. Combine that with helplessness, and the person can be left with deep-seated trauma.

Now let's return to adulthood. Say your boss comes down on you, and makes you feel like your job is at risk. And suddenly, your insecurities and self-doubt from when your mother used to belittle you become activated. Suddenly, your very survival is being threatened. What does the body do when its very survival is at risk? I'm sure you are familiar with adrenaline—the body's "superhuman" hormone that kicks in under times of duress. Adrenaline needs fuel. We are wired to survive imminent danger—but the first thing we need to do is pack in food for the long haul. Aka—binge!

My belief is that the binge is the body's way of surviving the threat on a primal, instinctive level, by fueling adrenaline. While stress eating reduces stress (temporarily) by temporarily creating feel-good endorphins, binging doesn't even need to taste good. In this state of being, any food will do; it just has to be a lot. In fact, it needs to be so much food that the brain actually needs to shut off, because, otherwise, you will stop eating too soon. The body is in total survival mode.

This is where our spirituality kicks in. Knowing that Hashem is perfect and that He loves you is essential. Remember that you are safe in His arms. Hashem, our Father in Heaven, is there for us always. He loves us more than the kindest father, and He takes care of us and keeps us safe. No harm can ever come to us because everything He does is perfect. It doesn't always feel perfect, and sometimes it feels very uncomfortable, but the discomfort is part of the perfection. Turn to Hashem, and ask Him for help in overcoming your fears and in realizing your worthiness. If you are someone who struggles with binge eating, working toward having this core belief system can be a tremendously helpful part of your recovery. My personal spiritual mentor is Gedale Fenster, and you can find his podcasts free on Spotify.

When you feel a binge coming on, commit to staying aware. Treat your binge like a mini-panic attack. Acknowledge the trigger that sets off the binges, and validate the perceived threat to your existence—out loud if possible. The goal is to help your brain understand that this is not a case of life and death and that your survival isn't actually threatened, even though it does feel like this at the moment. Stay present.

Stay conscious of your breathing and remind yourself that it is Hashem who is giving you each breath. You are safe and in good hands. You will survive and you will thrive.

On a practical note, a great way to stay present and not get lost in a binge is to track what you eat on a food log. The practice of being committed to writing down what you eat forces you to remain present. Thus, you will be less likely to go into a full-blown binge, because a real binge demands that you turn off your brain and go into a trance in order to continue eating. By staying present, your normal stop mechanisms will kick in before things get too out of hand.

BRAIN DRAIN

Stress eating and binge eating are dysfunctional and need to be eradicated.

BRAIN RETRAIN

Stress eating and binge eating are my body's ways of helping me survive a perceived threat. Both can be managed if I have the right perspective, as well as the right tools. I won't be afraid of my binges. I have the courage to face whatever my deeper fears are, knowing that I am safe in Hashem's hands.

31

HAVE A ROBUST TOOLKIT FOR EMOTIONAL REGULATION

I RECENTLY MET with a client who brought her baby along with her to our appointment. This is common in my practice, and my secretary is happy to keep an eye on a baby in a stroller while I meet with the mom in the room next door. About halfway through our session, the baby started to fuss a bit. The mother excused herself and ran to the reception area, handed her toddler a snack bag, and came back to resume our session.

"And," I thought to myself with a sigh, "this is where it all begins." The baby was in an unfamiliar environment, and couldn't see his mom. What he needed was Mom. What he got was a snack. And while the snack worked temporarily to calm him, it wasn't what he needed. His education in self-medicating with food was clearly already underway.

Once you become aware of it, you will notice that food is used in place of real emotional regulation all the time. Food is used to bribe, comfort, celebrate milestones, and numb pain from an early age. And it turns out—it works! If not for the unwanted side effects—weight gain, health problems, physical discomfort—food does a great job of temporarily getting us back to our homeostasis.

But does it really?

Picture a thirteen-year-old boy who mouths off to his dad. His dad slaps him across the face and sends him to his room. Now the boy is quiet. So, the sloppy, bullying parenting method must have worked, right? Of course not. Just because the kid shut up doesn't mean the parenting worked. It worked temporarily to silence the kid, but rest assured, this child hasn't learned anything, except maybe to slap his own child one day. He hasn't learned a thing, yet according to his dad, his parenting methods work.

Back to food. Yes, sweets and treats temporarily give us a jolt of pleasure and take away the discomfort of our emotional distress, but at what price? While there is a time and place for moderate amounts of stress eating (please refer to chapter 29, "Stress Eat Like a Professional"), it behooves us to cultivate a robust toolkit to emotionally regulate ourselves.

Come on a journey with me for a few minutes to a land with no food. In this land, we get our energy and nourishment from the sun. We still have family gatherings, *Yamim Tovim*, weddings, and *sheva berachos*, but food, and the desire for it, simply don't exist. How would you feel? Since food is one of the primary sources of pleasure for most people, a world like that might sound empty and lonely.

In a world as described above, how would you celebrate milestones? How would you relax after a stressful day? How would you connect with friends and family? Thinking in these terms affords us the realization that for many of us, food is so much more than nourishment. And while eating is meant to be both pleasurable and nourishing, for many of us it has become our primary source of pleasure, and for others, their only source.

If we can't picture relaxing, celebrating, de-stressing, or connecting with others without food in the picture, it has likely become our primary form of pleasure. This isn't necessarily an inherent problem, but for many people it becomes an issue as it begins to take its toll on their health and well-being.

If a world without food seems like a life not worth living, and if food has become your crutch or your drug, don't worry, you're not alone. And as far as I know, food hasn't been canceled, yet. But it is worth our while to try to cultivate a list of other ways to feel good that don't include food. Think about the two-year-old who totes his little blankie around wherever he goes. Think about how much relaxation, comfort, and pleasure he gets from that familiar little ragged piece of cloth. And picture a five-year-old who plays with his Legos and toys and escapes into a fantasy playland where he feels both safe and powerful. Imagine if we, as adults, had ways of feeling relaxed, comforted, safe, and powerful without food.

If you are spiritually connected, turning to your faith during times of physical discomfort can be a game changer. Turn to Hashem. Thank Him with sincere gratitude for all the good in your life. Thank Him for your eyes that see and your legs that work. Thank Him for your family, your friends, your job, and your house. Thank Him for your heat, your air-conditioning, your car, and the food in your fridge. And then ask for help.

Ask Him to help you through this moment of pain. Ask Him for strength to get through this food challenge. Ask Him for help with whatever other struggles you are facing. The pleasure of being connected to Hashem, the source of all good, can be the ultimate relief—the adult version of a child holding his blankie. If you do this as a daily practice, you will naturally be able to do this during your times of discomfort and struggle.

If one doesn't feel that they are in a spiritually connected place or are working on it but aren't there yet, they can usually find other things that bring them pleasure. We tend not to utilize them too often, as food is readily available, and the effect is almost instantaneous. A hot shower, playing silly games with a toddler, a walk around the block, a call to a funny friend, an adult coloring book, a funny video clip, flipping through an old photo album, giving someone a compliment or a hug, getting a hug—the list goes on and on.

Try to make a list of ways that you would find relaxing, connecting, and comforting that don't involve food, and practice utilizing them so that you'll learn to trust them and they become your "go to."

Please note: Do not include items on your list just because they are popular. For example, I literally hate baths; I find them boring, claustrophobic, and icky. But on lots of these self-care lists, it's way up there. Regardless, it isn't going on *my* list.

BRAIN DRAIN

I need food to have fun, relax, de-stress, and comfort myself.

BRAIN RETRAIN

Food is one tool to accomplish the above, but I have other tools in my toolkit.

32

GET COMFORTABLE BEING UNCOMFORTABLE

IT'S CHILLY INSIDE, so you put on a sweater. You have a headache, so you pop some Advil. You feel jealous of a friend, so you make some snide remarks to cut her down a notch and make yourself feel better. Basic human behavior. We live in a pretty cushy world—one that has trained us to believe that life should always be comfortable, and all discomfort should be immediately resolved.

But what if we rethink that? What if we come to the realization that not all discomfort is bad and needs to be immediately resolved? What if we got comfortable feeling uncomfortable?

My husband and I recently visited some family friends on a cold winter night in Philadelphia. Our family was invited to a neighbor's house for a dinner party, and we chose to walk the few blocks rather than piling ourselves into the car. It was a bitter, cold night, with icy winds cutting into us, and most of us were somewhat underdressed, as we hadn't anticipated walking. As my husband and I huddled in our coats and shivered our way down the block, I noticed that the host, dressed in a light windbreaker, was walking briskly and comfortably with his arms loosely by his side. This was in stark contrast to my family's huddled, whiny, shivery trudging.

When I asked our host why he seemed so obnoxiously comfortable while we were all suffering and willing the walk to be over, he answered simply, yet profoundly, "I practice the teachings of Buddhism. I have trained myself to resist nothing. Resisting something only gives it more power. Yes, I am uncomfortable, but I embrace the sensations and embrace the moment I am in."

The concepts of "resist nothing" and "embrace discomfort" are in direct contrast to the general American way most of us are partial to: if something is uncomfortable, make it go away.

When we have an urge to eat more than planned, let's try to sit with that urge or feeling for a bit. Acknowledge it, notice the discomfort, identify where it is in your body, maybe even rate it on a scale of one to ten, but don't do anything about it. Don't fight it or will it away, don't distract yourself, and definitely don't eat to make it go away. Accept it.

In accepting it, you will find that if the urge was just a craving, it will take about twenty minutes and then pass on its own. As you practice this quiet acceptance, you will build up your tolerance for physical or emotional discomfort.

This is, *l'havdil*, aligned with the teachings of Rebbe Nachman of Breslov, whose lessons have recently become a major influence on me. Rebbe Nachman teaches that when we resist pain and discomfort, we actually give it more power and more energy over us. When we embrace the pain and discomfort, we are able to face it head-on.

Pain is not a mistake or an evolutionary accident. Pain is a message, a tool designed to help us grow. By masking it or numbing it with food, we completely miss the message and will have to relearn the lesson at a later date. If we are uncomfortable and we numb that discomfort with food, we are now left with two problems—the original problem that brought about the physical discomfort, as well as the secondary problem, the extra weight we need to lose and the feelings of guilt and regret that come with it.

Of course, this is not referring to legitimate hunger. If you are legitimately hungry, it's usually because it is time to eat. Please go ahead and eat the next scheduled food on your plan. But when you are well fed and not overly stressed but are still feeling the urge to eat, there is usually an underlying uneasiness that has nothing to do with food that requires your attention. If you have taken some measures to reduce your stress and are still feeling uncomfortable, try embracing the discomfort. It is there to help. Don't resist it. Embrace the discomfort, and perhaps try to figure out what is really bothering you.

BRAIN DRAIN

When I have an urge to eat, I feel physically or emotionally uncomfortable, so I have to eat to make it go away.

BRAIN RETRAIN

It's okay to be uncomfortable, sometimes. I can handle it, and, in fact, it is good for me and has the potential to help me grow. I don't have to do anything about it or make it go away. It will pass on its own.

33

KNOW WHEN TO HOLD 'EM AND WHEN TO FOLD

IF YOU ARE FEELING a bit confused right now, I apologize. We have gone through several different scenarios, and in each one, I have given what could be perceived as contradictory advice. Avoid temptation. Respect your hunger. Build up your resistance by treating cravings like a tantrum. Learn to sit with your discomfort. Embrace stress eating and give in. But just a little. How are you supposed to know which tool applies to which situation?

Honestly, there is no single right answer. The tool you use is up to you, and different times will call for different tools. But I will try to break things down for you so that you can have a starting point and make an informed decision.

Here are a few basic guidelines. But first, we need to determine where the urge to eat is coming from. Check in with your stomach first. And check the clock. If you haven't eaten in two to three hours, you are likely legitimately hungry. This is not to say that you aren't also stressed or tempted by food that isn't on plan, but when mixed with hunger, we are suddenly in dangerous territory. If you determine that you are hungry, eat.

A good way to determine if you are actually hungry is to pay attention to what you want to eat. If you are willing to eat pretty much anything, this is likely real hunger, and you should eat some food. The best choice would be to eat the next item on your plan or to eat some filling low-calorie protein such as yogurt or a few extra ounces of chicken.

Once you have taken care of your hunger, you can use the following guidelines:

- If you are in a situation where you are neither stressed nor hungry but, rather, being pulled by food because it looks tempting or others around you are eating it, I would recommend practicing your resistance techniques: Notice the HUT, acknowledge it, and make a power move to end the battle.
- If you can remove yourself from the situation, or alternatively, remove the food, do so. If you can't leave the room or can't get rid of the food, I don't find that being in a prolonged battle is a good idea, as it usually doesn't end well. Even if you end up resisting, studies have found that you will feel so emotionally depleted by utilizing so much self-control that you will end up going overboard and giving in later on. Rather, have a small taste of whatever is calling your name, enjoy it, and be done with it.
- If you notice that the urge to eat is coming from somewhere other than your stomach—such as from your chest or your jaw—it is likely stress-related. In this case, you should use your emotional eating tools. Have a small amount of stress-reducing food, and then move on to the other tools in your toolkit.
- If you have already done some stress eating and have already tried some other forms of stress reduction, but are still feeling the urge to eat, I would suggest trying to work on sitting with the discomfort and work on being okay with it.

BRAIN DRAIN

I don't know which tool to use—I am probably doing this wrong.

BRAIN RETRAIN

All the tools above are appropriate at different times, but using any of them is better than using none of them. I will go ahead and trust my judgment, and if I get it wrong, recalibrate for the next time. The only mistakes are the ones I don't learn from.

34

DON'T BE LIKE HARRY HOUDINI

HAVE YOU EVER HEARD of Harry Houdini, the famous Hungarian-born American illusionist and stunt performer, noted for his daring escape acts? His most famous acts included freeing himself from handcuffs, chains, and ropes, and he was famous not only for his incredible skill but also for his unmatched strength and stamina.

One day, after one of his major performances, a fan by the name of J. Gordon Whitehead came to visit Harry in his dressing room and asked him if the rumors about his incredible strength were true. Houdini casually replied in the affirmative. Whitehead then delivered a couple of strong punches to Harry's gut. Unfortunately, these punches ultimately caused Harry severe appendicitis, and he died shortly afterward, in the prime of his life.

How was the strongest man in the world brought down by a couple of punches to the stomach? What went wrong? Witnesses reported that Houdini was reclining on a couch at the time of the encounter, having broken his ankle while performing several days earlier. They reported that Houdini winced at each blow and stopped Whitehead suddenly in the midst of a punch, gesturing that he had had enough. It was later confirmed that Harry had not had the opportunity to prepare himself against the blows, as he had not expected Whitehead to strike him so suddenly and forcefully. In short, Harry had been caught off-guard and hadn't had a chance to set his muscles to prepare for the blows. And shortly afterward he was dead.

My point here is simple. When we are prepared for a situation, we can set ourselves up for success. When we aren't prepared, we can expect to get sucker-punched in the gut. Of course, for me, this relates directly back to our food plans. Knowing what events, scenarios, and situations are coming up and planning for our version of a successful outcome is a critical component of our long-term weight loss success.

I always tell my clients that if every day of the year looked like a random Tuesday in February, dieting would likely be simple. We would get into a routine that works, stick to a schedule that works, and repeat it until it's as habitual as flossing our teeth. Okay, let's be honest; some of us forget to floss. But at least as habitual as brushing our teeth.

But life isn't like that. We have Shabbos, Yom Tov, birthday parties, and graduations. We have weddings, shiva houses, and vacations. We have snow days, sick days, and endless *simchahs*, *baruch Hashem*. We have days when we are running errands for nine hours straight and days when our tire goes flat and our kids stay home sick. While we can't plan for every eventuality, we can definitely prepare for most of them.

But oftentimes, we don't take the few minutes to set ourselves up for success, and before we know it, we are lost in the fudge brownies, telling ourselves our diet starts tomorrow—but for real this time! Let's not be like Harry Houdini, getting sucker-punched in the gut. Let's stop underestimating the importance of being prepared.

BRAIN DRAIN

I was out all day and now I am starving. I'll just grab a few chips and a chocolate bar. Tomorrow, I will get back on track.

BRAIN RETRAIN

I am going to be out for several hours tomorrow. Let me pack a lunch, so I don't come home starving and make a mess of things when I get home like I did last week. Life is more predictable than we think. I will plan for success.

35

NO, THE VACATION ISN'T OVER, AND YOU AREN'T DONE BAKING

OFTENTIMES, when clients walk into the office after a vacation or a baking marathon having gained a couple of pounds, they are visibly embarrassed and announce sheepishly, "Thank God that's over—I was really a disaster. But now I am ready to get back on track."

While I admire the enthusiasm, and love that they are firing on all cylinders, I usually try to give them a bit of a reality check. You may be done baking for Yom Tov, but unless you are planning on dying in the next couple of weeks, there will be many more baking marathons coming your way. And before hitting the ground running, it is worth our while to take a couple of minutes to reflect on how things went—both positively and negatively, and how you feel about it.

I encourage my clients to have a broader lens when it comes to weight management. Rather than committing to a fresh start for the upcoming week, let's get a perspective on your vacation habits, Erev Shabbos and Shabbos habits, Yom Tov habits, baking habits, etc. Let's reflect for a few minutes on what went well, so we can repeat that next time, and what didn't go quite as well, so we can be better prepared for that next time. Because while we may be ready to hit the ground running, the situation that messed us up will reappear at some point down the line. Guaranteed. Next time, let's get it right!

Of course, sometimes, there's nothing to reflect upon. I had a client who returned from a five-star, all-inclusive vacation having gained six pounds over the course of ten days. She came back into my office ready to rock and roll, and when I asked her to reflect, she told me she had zero regrets. She enjoyed every bite and understood that this ten-day trip was a once-in-a-lifetime experience that she would likely never have again. She had enjoyed living in the moment and wasn't disturbed by her weight gain. I respect that.

But, in general, instead of being myopic, it pays to take a broader look and reflect on how we would like to see this situation play out in the future. If a client just finished her baking marathon and was nibbling on cake and cookies throughout the entire time until she felt physically ill, I would ask her what might have helped.

Clients often come up with great ideas; here are some examples:

- Baking smaller batches more often so it doesn't feel as rare and, therefore, excusable.
- Baking earlier in the day when self-control is still a viable option.
- Leaving cut-up vegetables on the counter to nibble on while baking.
- Packaging everything up and freezing it immediately.
- Asking a family member to check in on me to see how I'm doing with my commitment to resistance.
- Baking things that are delicious but not the most tempting.
- Allowing myself one or two small portions at the end of the day.

All these are great ideas, and I am sure you can come up with some of your own.

The point is not to see these non-routine events as one-time things, but as ongoing, predictable, and plan-for-able challenges. In other words, even the non-routine days have an element of predictability to them, and if we reflect a bit, we can be better prepared for the next time. Developing the skills needed for the non-routine but ongoing challenges takes a little bit more effort and foresight, but it's not impossible.

If twenty out of fifty-two weeks a year are non-routine and we gain a couple pounds during each of those weeks, we spend the other thirty-two weeks undoing the damage and will have a difficult time gaining any real momentum. Let's not give our weeks away so readily. If twenty weeks a year are non-routine and we are well prepared and pretty much manage to maintain our weight, the other thirty-two weeks are ours to make some serious progress.

Your baking marathon may have ended, but your baking career is still going strong—and since hindsight is twenty-twenty, let's use it to our advantage. The past informs our future.

> **BRAIN DRAIN**
> Yom Tov season is over. I was a total disaster, but I'm ready to get back on track.
>
> **BRAIN RETRAIN**
> This Yom Tov season is over, but I'm going to take a few minutes to reflect, so that next Yom Tov season leaves me feeling proud.

36
DIET DERAILERS

IF YOU HAVE a Diet Derailer in your life, this chapter is for you. You know who diet derailers are. It's the mother-in-law who insists that you taste her latest recipe because she made it especially for you. It's the friend you meet with for brunch who tells you she's concerned that you might have an eating disorder even though you are far from your goal weight. It's the husband who brings home chocolate as a surprise, despite knowing that you are being careful to stick to what you committed to doing.

Most of us tend to eat the quiche being offered just to keep the mother-in-law happy, choose poorly at brunch to placate the jealous friend, and eat the chocolate because, well, it's chocolate. And we don't want to insult our husbands.

What's missing here, of course, is boundaries. Setting boundaries means stating your needs and following through, even if it might make someone uncomfortable in the process. Let's just clarify this a bit.

Setting boundaries isn't the same thing as being rude. Telling your mother-in-law that you would love some quiche but that you are working hard to stick to your food plan is boundary setting. Telling her she's an overbearing shrew and also a terrible cook is rude. Telling your friend that you would prefer an egg-white omelet over the seven-cheese quesadilla she's pushing you to order is boundary setting. Telling her to take a look in the mirror and pointing out that it wouldn't kill her to eat an egg-white omelet once in a while is rude. Thanking your husband profusely for thinking of you and mentioning that fresh cut fruit would be even more appreciated is boundary setting. Throwing the chocolate in the trash while he is still standing there is rude.

Why is boundary setting, especially when it comes to our diets, so difficult for us? Like I mentioned before, boundary setting often makes the other person uncomfortable. Your mother-in-law might feel hurt and rejected; your friend might feel jealous or uncomfortable with her food choices; and your husband might be slightly disappointed. Again, they don't have to feel that way, and they can choose not to feel that way. But they likely *will* feel that way because we can't protect them from their own humanness.

Remember—it's not your job to make sure that no one ever feels any negative feelings. Many of us have been trained from when we are young to put other people's feelings first, but this becomes unhealthy when it's at the expense of our own needs.

Let's play it out. Say your mother-in-law is plying you with her world-famous cherry pie. You grab the opportunity to set some boundaries, and you say, "Thanks, Mom, that looks delicious, but I ate enough already. I am really trying to stay disciplined here. But it definitely looks tempting!" She pushes back with, "Well, I worked really hard on it, and I made it especially for you because I know you love this recipe—just try a little bit."

Now, you are torn because if you don't eat the pie, she's going to feel bad, and then you are going to feel bad that you made her feel bad. And if you do eat the pie, you know you will regret it later. Well, guess what—you did not make her feel bad! She can choose to brush it off, be understanding, be insulted, or be any number of things—that's her stuff. In fact, if she could be gracious about it, this situation would be a whole lot easier.

The only thing you can control in this scenario is how you behave and how you feel. I am here to tell you that the only problem in this entire scenario is you. You feel bad that she feels hurt. And then you are upset that she's making you feel bad by feeling bad. Well, how about just don't feel bad?

This is the crux of boundary setting. We avoid setting boundaries because there's usually some fallout. Someone is left feeling hurt, and you feel uncomfortable for making them feel uncomfortable. You give in, but it comes at a cost. Of course, when there's food involved, it's even a bit trickier because there's that part of you that secretly wants an excuse to give in and eat the pie or the chocolate, and would love to justify it with, "Well, I didn't want to insult my husband." I mean, is there any better justification than that?

The good news is that boundary setting gets easier with practice—just like everything else. It's empowering to politely advocate for yourself without worrying about the fallout. And it's even more emboldening to do so in the face of temptation when your inner chocoholic is begging for a fix. Give it a try, but remember, not everyone is going to love you for it, and you may not even love you for it. You may end up feeling bad for making someone else feel bad. But do it anyway. You can blame me if you need to. You do you, Boo.

BRAIN DRAIN

When my family members push me to eat, I feel bad insulting them, so I just give in.

BRAIN RETRAIN

As long as I state my needs politely and appropriately, I don't have to worry about how others might feel or react. Sometimes, boundary setting won't feel very good, but I'm okay with that because my needs are important.

37

BRIBERY 101

IF YOU ARE struggling to stick to your commitments, it might be time to try some external motivation, aka bribery. The problem with adult bribery is that it works differently from children's bribery. Children's bribery is simple: if you don't get kicked out of math class, you will get a quarter when you come home (based on a true story circa sixth grade—twenty-five cents was a lot of money back then!).

The rules for bribing kids are simple—offer them something they wouldn't otherwise have access to, strike a deal with them, and watch the magic unfold. Adults, however, are slightly trickier to bribe. How many times have you told yourself, "If I lose ten pounds, I will treat myself to a massage, or, if I lose twenty pounds, I'll take that vacation to Miami," only to find yourself going for the massage anyway and taking the vacation regardless of weight loss success. Because we have access to our own funds, we pretty much do what we want to do.

How do we, as adults, bribe ourselves? Is it even possible? The answer is simple—to quote Dave Ramsey, use OPM, Other People's Money. (He is talking about something completely different—I'm just borrowing his phraseology, but it's way out of context.) When it comes to OPM, we are willing to do a lot for very little, kind of exactly the way it was when we were kids.

There was a stage in my life when I was having a hard time getting myself to bed on time. I would stay up well past 2:00 a.m. browsing Zillow, catching up on non-essential WhatsApps, and generally wasting time until my eyes burned and my brain was exploding. Then I would caffeinate my way through the next day, which, of course, led to more restlessness the following night. I was a zombie. My work, my family, and my body were suffering, but I couldn't get myself out of this cycle. I promised myself the world if I would only get to bed on time. And I gave myself everything I promised. But I still kept going to bed after 2:00 a.m.

Finally, I discussed it with my mom. "You know what I need?" I told her. "I need one of those bedtime charts I had when I was little. I need you to give me five dollars for every night that I get to bed before midnight." My mom, always my greatest cheerleader, graciously agreed. And for five dollars, I got myself to bed by midnight. Simple as that. All I needed was that little bit of external motivation, and it couldn't be done from my budget—it had to be extra.

I see this with my clients all the time. They leave my office intending to track their food or prepare lunch or drink their water, and week after week, they come back telling me the reasons why it didn't work out for them. But when I offer them a five-dollar credit to be used toward future nutrition consultations if they stick to their commitments, suddenly they are on a mission.

The psychology behind this is basic. Bribery works. The problem is only when we are playing with our own money, because then it isn't really bribery so much as it is a reshuffling of the already accessible funds. For it to be bribery, and for it to work, figure out how to access OPM. Find someone who loves you and cares about you with whom you don't share money, and see if you can get that person to bribe you.

Note of caution: For this strategy to be most effective, it is best not to link the bribe to an amount of weight lost, but, rather, to a behavior. For example, instead of having your sister pay you three dollars for every pound you lose, have your sister give you twenty-five cents for every cup of water you drink or one dollar for every day that you complete your food log. Because the scale is affected by many factors and isn't always under our control, but our behaviors are.

BRAIN DRAIN

Bribery doesn't work on me—I have tried it. I just end up giving myself what I want without actually sticking to my commitment.

BRAIN RETRAIN

I'm going to go ahead and give it another try, but I'm going to make sure I am doing it effectively. Commitment and accountability may take creativity and ingenuity.

PART III

KEEPING IT OFF

38

FLASHES OF INSPIRATION

IT'S TIME TO REVISIT a topic that we began in chapter 16, but this time from a different angle and in more depth.

While almost all of my clients start off strong and committed, I often notice that after a couple of months, or, in some cases, sooner, the weight loss will start to taper off, the food logs will be spotty, and they will seem a bit discouraged. When I ask them about it, they will usually tell me that they are no longer as desperate as they were in the beginning and, therefore, no longer as motivated.

This is super normal. In fact, I have come to see it as part of the weight loss journey. Most of us are familiar with that new diet "rush." We finally decide to take control of our weight and choose a plan, eager to follow it to a T. Desperate to lose the extra pounds and high from the feeling of being back in control, things usually start off strong. But eventually, something comes along and sets us back. And suddenly the adrenaline-fueled rush seems to dissipate, and our old habits come creeping back. This is normal.

Previously, we dealt with why this happens and the first step to handling this discouragement, which validates the experience. I remind my clients that the honeymoon doesn't last forever, and eventually, as desperation dissipates, so does the inspiration.

Then comes the follow-up conversation—and the point of this chapter—how do we get our motivation back? I ask my clients to think about other experiences in which they had a momentary flash of inspiration. Say you were driving recklessly and almost lost control of your car. You are shaken to the core and swear you will never drive over 60 mph again. And for weeks you remember that fear of almost dying, and you drive like a little old lady on her way to church. But a few months later, you notice that your speed limit has picked up a bit, and a few weeks after that, you find yourself rushing to the airport and pushing 70 mph. (Okay, let's be honest, it was closer to 90 mph.) How do I get my inspiration back? How do I ensure that I don't slip back into my reckless driving habits?

The honest answer? By understanding that we can't always be fueled by inspiration. Like we said, inspiration comes and goes in flashes. And the last thing we want is another near-accident to remotivate us. What can we do to ensure our safe driving? Ready for the answer? It may not be alluring or exciting, but the answer is taking your inspiration and turning it into unwavering commitment.

If I am truly committed to driving safely, whether I feel like it or not, whether I'm rushing or not, whether I'm at risk of crashing or not, I must be willing to implement whatever it takes to develop this habit and this discipline. Maybe it means I'll install a speed tracker and send the report to my husband each night. Maybe it means that for every mile per hour I drive above the speed limit, I donate one dollar to charity. Maybe it means that I have to take Ubers for a week if I speed, even if I don't get caught. I can't expect to always be inspired, but I can ensure that I am always committed. And while inspiration comes and goes, inspiration can be used to put a set of rules and accountability in place to keep me in check when I am less inspired.

When clients come in discouraged that they aren't as motivated as they once were, I welcome them to Stage 2 of the weight loss journey—the part that's not fueled by adrenaline or desperation but by rock-solid commitment and the systems of support and accountability needed to follow through on those commitments.

Here are some things to commit to while you are feeling inspired:

- Commit to tracking your food in a food log.
- Commit to planning for upcoming challenges.
- Commit to preparing your food.

- Commit to keeping your fridge and pantry well stocked and removing triggers.
- Commit to weekly accountability with a friend or coach.
- Commit to reflecting and troubleshooting when things don't go well.

The beautiful thing about holding ourselves accountable to our commitment is that we ensure consistent repetition. And consistent repetition creates habits. And habits become more and more deeply ingrained, until they are almost second nature. Which means that while the weight loss struggle may not get easier, we get stronger.

The first step may be desperation and inspiration, which breeds temporary success. But when harnessed properly, we develop commitment and accountability—which breeds real and lasting habit change.

> BRAIN DRAIN
>
> I started out so strong—where did my motivation go? I can't do this anymore! It's just too hard.
>
> BRAIN RETRAIN
>
> If I stay committed to my new behaviors even when it's tough, they will become habits and will no longer feel as difficult. Grit and stamina are key.

39

PERCEPTION VS. REALITY: AM I REALLY THE ONLY ONE WORKING THIS HARD?

HAVE YOU EVER FELT that you are the only one who has to work hard to maintain a healthy body weight, while "everyone else" gets to "eat whatever they want" without gaining an ounce? Instagram, WhatsApp statuses, Facebook, and other forms of social media are all great ways to promote the belief that everyone out there is living her best life except you. And, of course, they all have beach houses, designer clothes, perfect spouses, and perfect teeth.

Here are some more common perceptions that are patently false:

- Once I decide to lose weight, the process should be quick and smooth.
- I used to eat even more than this when I was younger and never had an issue, so why should there be an issue now?
- I am working harder than everyone else. It's really not fair.
- I know I went off plan, but I shouldn't have gained that much.

Let's break this down a bit. First of all, not everyone is partying. Take a closer look around. Some people aren't eating at all. Some people are partying but are quite overweight. Some people are partying and are thin, but you don't know if this was the only time that they ate all day. And some people are headed home to take a handful of laxatives to purge what they just ate. And others have been dieting hard up until this moment, knowing that this party or event is special and worthwhile enough to indulge a bit.

Think about the people you know who eat whatever they want whenever they want and still maintain a slim figure. You probably can come up with one or two right off the bat. But if you try to list a few more, you will probably draw a blank. Our tunnel vision allows us to see only what we want to see—that we are somehow much more deprived than the people around us. But if we widen our lens and take a closer look, we see the actual truth.

This reminds me of one of my very first clients, who happens to be my sister. My sister Elana got married when she was nineteen years old. At her wedding she was five feet, seven inches and weighed 125 pounds. Ten months later (and two weeks overdue), she clocked in at over 205 pounds. Yes, she had gained over eighty pounds during her pregnancy. She came to me a few weeks postpartum, determined to regain her figure. I worked with her for months, coaching and cheering her on. About seven months postpartum, she was about ten pounds away from her realistic goal weight of 135 pounds. Phew!

Throughout the process, I encouraged Elana to treat herself with her favorite foods here and there, so that she wouldn't feel deprived. But she was so determined to lose the weight that she kept pushing off this planned treat; she really didn't need it. She decided when she reached 140 pounds she would have a cheese Danish—her favorite treat.

And that's exactly what happened. A couple weeks later, only a few pounds away from her goal weight, we all gathered together for a family party. As planned, Elana sat down with a cheese Danish the size of a small continent, ready to enjoy her well-deserved treat. Just then, a more distant relative walked by and commented to her, "You are so lucky you get to eat whatever you want and still lose weight."

Elana and I both looked at each other and burst out laughing. *Whatever I want, yeah right.* She had been so disciplined for months, and this well-deserved, well-planned treat was a long time coming. But to an outsider who wasn't privy to the months of preparation, planning, discipline, self-control, and habit building, it certainly appeared that my sister was one of those lucky people who ate whatever she wanted and stayed thin.

The problem with these flawed expectations is that when we feel that we are working harder than we should be or harder than others, we lose our motivation.

I recently attended a food show to promote my line of health food products. When I discovered that the show was taking place at the Meadowlands in New Jersey, less than fifteen minutes from my house, I was thrilled. No long drive, and no traffic—what could be better? I left the house thirty minutes early to leave time for parking and set out for a fun day of networking (and food tasting).

Unfortunately, I missed a turn and then another, and before I knew it, forty minutes were added to my ETA. I felt my blood pressure rise and my frustration start to mount. This was supposed to be easy. And I left early. And now I'm running late. And I don't even know how I missed that turn, so I may make the exact same mistake again.

As I drove, though, I was struck by a realization. The reason I was so frustrated was because my expectation was that this would be easy. Had I been driving to Manhattan, I would have left my house earlier and been even more prepared, and I would have been less frustrated if something went wrong.

It was my expectation that this trip would be easy that made the whole experience infuriating. I realized that this is often how it is with dieting. When we are tempted by foods that are not on plan, we rationalize tasting some, telling ourselves, "A little bit won't hurt." We simply don't feel that resisting twenty-five or fifty calories of food is worth the effort that it takes to resist it. It feels like too much work for something so small. And when we don't lose as quickly as we should, we quickly get discouraged and give up on the process.

Let me tell you a little secret. Dieting isn't easy. It's hard for almost everyone. More than half of American women are overweight or obese, and most of those women are trying. So yes, sticking to a food plan and exercising self-discipline is difficult, but not just for you—for pretty much everyone with a pulse and a small intestine.

BRAIN DRAIN

Everyone is partying, while I'm sitting here struggling to lose each pound.

BRAIN RETRAIN

It may seem like everyone is partying and losing weight, but in reality, most people are struggling mightily to keep a healthy body weight. I am likely not seeing the whole picture. As Gedale Fenster has been known to say, "Stay in your lane."

40

RICH OR POOR? TALL OR SHORT?

SOMETIMES, when clients have a particularly challenging week, they come to their appointments super excited to get on the scale and see the fruits of their labor. "I worked really hard this week—I'd better have lost weight!" And more often than not, not only did they not lose any weight, but they may have even gained a bit. And, of course, they are disappointed and frustrated having worked so hard "for nothing."

I try to remind my clients that if they compare their food intake to what they could have eaten, they deserve a gold medal because there was so much temptation around. But if they compare their food intake to what they usually eat on their plan, they definitely ate more. I console them by reminding them that the scale doesn't dictate whether or not they were successful, and if they were proud of their choices and decisions, they still deserve that gold medal. But navigating a challenging week successfully doesn't necessarily mean losing weight. Because hard is relative.

For as long as I can remember, I defined my looks first by my height. I was the tallest in my class by the time I was in fifth grade, and had grown to my full height of five feet, nine inches by the time I was in seventh grade. I remember an incident where I got kicked out of the classroom for some misdemeanor and was sent to wait in the hallway, presumably until I somehow magically learned to behave. Of course, while I was out there my principal appeared, and started lecturing me. Just then, my teacher stepped out to invite me back in, and I will never forget the image of the two of them wagging their fingers up at me, chins tilted up, as I towered above them trying to stifle my giggles.

Fast forward about ten years later. I was newly married, and I took a trip with my husband to Amsterdam. As we took in all the sights and smells, I noticed something startling. I was surrounded by six-foot, blonde women looking very much like me. For the first time in my life, I felt what average felt like. It was so disorienting. I was no longer the tall blonde girl—many of the women were much taller (and blonder!).

I came to the clear realization that absolutely everything is relative—a matter of perspective—and really depends on what is being compared. I am probably rich compared to most of the people in Africa, and statistically, even as compared to most people in the world, but when I go to the Hamptons in the summer, I am relatively poor. I might have the nicest car on my little cul-de-sac, but the same car would be considered slightly embarrassing when pulling up to my cousin's place on Long Island.

I like to share this perspective with my clients when they tell me they are frustrated by their results after working really hard. Sure, dieting is a struggle for many, but it's relative to the environment in which you find yourself. If you had a week of work events and birthday parties, you may have worked very hard to stay on plan so that it wouldn't translate into extra weight loss on the scale.

One of my busier offices is in a building that has a gourmet supermarket on the ground floor. Inside that supermarket is an artisanal chocolate shop called The Nuttery. The Nuttery is filled with hand-crafted milk chocolate delicacies that are known throughout the neighborhood to induce chocolate comas and death by chocolate.

I sit with my clients and tell them, "If this office was five flights down, in The Nuttery, I would want a gold medal for every day that I came home from work without indulging. And I would expect my weight loss to reflect that battle as well! Nothing less than a two-pound weight loss per hour for my Herculean efforts to resist would be acceptable. However, sitting here snugly in my office five flights up, the chocolate is pretty much irrelevant."

Except, of course, when I start talking about it and then start dreaming about it.

My clients get my drift—hard work is relative to the context and doesn't always translate into weight loss. This doesn't mean that we should never go to parties or to restaurants; it just means that we should expect to work harder than usual and at the same time expect less weight loss than usual. And that's okay—not every week is a weight loss week. Some weeks are skill-building weeks, and those are just as valuable in the big picture.

BRAIN DRAIN

I worked so hard to practice self-control at that party, and it was all for nothing. This isn't working.

BRAIN RETRAIN

Working harder doesn't always mean losing more. But hard work is what fuels skill building and ultimately builds new habits. I will keep my expectations in check and understand that hard work is relative.

41

IF YOU ARE BORED, IT MIGHT BE BECAUSE YOU ARE BORING

DON'T TAKE THIS the wrong way. I am not trying to say that you are boring as a person, but often, when clients report that they are having trouble sticking to their food plan because they are bored of their food, it is usually not the diet that's the problem, but them. They just aren't being very interesting.

I usually challenge my clients to tell me what they would want to eat if they weren't on a diet. Because I never recommend cutting out full food groups or even specific foods, my clients know that they can pretty much have any food they want in moderation. Remember the key word here is food—junk food doesn't count. And obviously, the other key word is moderation. But when posed with the offer to tell me what they want to eat, my clients often draw a blank.

When I review their food logs, I always see some version of the following: salmon, tuna, eggs, chicken breast, repeat. Well, how about some whitefish, pollack, sea bass, or even lox instead of the usual salmon? How about you swap that chicken breast out for some duck, lamb, turkey, or bison? How about having a variety of vegetables other than lettuce, tomatoes, and cucumbers in your salad?

When's the last time you switched up your spices? One cannot exist on onion powder, garlic powder, salt, and pepper forever. Take a walk down the spice aisle, and you will find over four hundred different spices begging for your attention. And what about changing your cooking method? If you eat grilled chicken for seven weeks in a row, of course you are bored. Try poaching, broiling, steaming, or smoking your food, and you will feel like you are eating something brand new.

Another way to keep the food from feeling boring is to improve the presentation. Please don't eat your sandwich off a plastic plate or, even worse, still half-wrapped in foil. Get some pretty dishes and spend thirty seconds on the plating and presentation, and you will feel like you just had something brand new. According to a 2012 Cornell University study published in the *Journal of Consumer Research*, eating off darker-colored dishes leaves you more satisfied than eating off lighter-colored ones—who knew?

Also, may I suggest that you set up a rotation? Don't eat eggs every single morning until you can't look an egg in the face again. If you have some healthy protein pancakes on Sunday, an omelet on Monday, overnight oats on Tuesday, a protein smoothie on Wednesday, a bowl of whole grain cereal with milk on Thursday, whole wheat French toast on Friday, and a low-calorie muffin on Saturday, I would venture to say that by Sunday you will be ready to look those eggs in the eye again. If you are only having something once a week, it can take years before you are sick of it.

BRAIN DRAIN

I can't stick to my food plan long term because I am already getting bored of it.

BRAIN RETRAIN

All foods are okay in moderation, so my food plan isn't boring. But I might be. I'll put in a bit more effort because it's important to me.

42

THE TUG-OF-WAR

AS YOU CONTINUE on your weight loss journey, there may be some frustration. You may have some trouble sticking to your plan, and *Yamim Tovim* may keep you at a temporary standstill—expected, but still frustrating—and your progress may be slower than you anticipated.

And then comes along a well-meaning friend or even a Google ad touting the brand-new best-selling vitamin, powder, pill, or injection that promises speedy and permanent weight loss. Yup, Google knows you are on a diet. Or you hear a story about a neighbor or family member who lost eight pounds in one week doing the New Green Lean Machine diet, or the Shake and Cake Diet, or the Boil and Toil diet, and suddenly, your resolve goes out the window. It can feel pretty silly that all you lost in three months is ten pounds, when your cousin lost almost that much in three days.

You start to question if all this is even worth it. There must be a faster way! Little secret—of course there is. And not only that, but you've likely tried it, or some version of it, already. Because there are endless ways to repackage the quick fix. Just starve for a couple days or weeks and voilà! The weight comes off. The problem is that all the quick fixes that are out there are temporary, and you know from past experience, the weight always comes back.

Alright, you say, I'll take temporary. But I'll be smarter than everyone else. I'll do the quick fix for a week or two and drop five or ten pounds, and then ease right back into this program. My friend, let me tell you:

that's the oldest story in the book. The problem is that every time you eat too little, your body will fight back, and it will win.

When the body is deprived, threatened, or undernourished, it perceives that food is scarce. Our body is wired to protect us against dying of hunger. It is much more concerned with survival than with you fitting into your skinny jeans. As soon as the opportunity presents itself, you will be faced with an uncontrollable biological urge to replenish your fat storage and energy reserves.

Imagine it in these terms. It's like saying I will sleep for three hours a night for a week straight and then ease into seven hours a night. No chance in France. Your body will first need to crash at some point and recover fully by oversleeping before getting onto a seven-hour sleep schedule, despite all your intentions.

In other words, sugar and carbs will hunt you down, find you, and stick to you, no matter how determined and well-intentioned you are. It may be at the end of the week, or after the 30 Days to Skinny are over, or at some other time in the near future, but at some point, the body will restore itself to its former levels of fat reserves.

The only way to avoid this phenomenon is to lose the weight in a way that doesn't threaten the body—slowly and steadily, without drastic measures and without cutting out full food groups. Trust me—there's no way around, only through. And if you do decide to go the quick-fix route, in the end, you will have lost nothing but time. And for those of you that have been through the cycle before, it'll be another depressing episode that batters your self-esteem, and makes you feel like it's your fault or that you have no self-control, when really it's basic biology. Spare yourself.

This is one end of the rope—the urge to hurry things along by taking the shortcut or quick-fix route. On the other end of the rope is the opposite extreme. While we plug away at the pounds and rewire our brains, we can often despair at the pace of the process and want to just give it all up. "I'm still so fat; I might as well eat," is a common refrain that I hear in my office. Every setback and every challenge leave us wondering if we should just give up.

To this, I advise that unless you are planning to give up forever, which I doubt is the case, it would be silly to quit now. Chances are that even if you do give up now, at some point, you will decide to watch what you are eating again. And when that happens, you will be left with more weight to lose, and it'll be more depressing and overwhelming than it is right now. Push through the discouragement, perhaps even treat yourself to something extra, but do not give in to the little voice compelling you to quit. Don't trust that voice—it's going to change its mind eventually.

Being aware of the tug-of-war that pulls at us from both sides from time to time (or all the time) will allow us to keep fighting and stay the course, without being swayed to go the quick-fix route, and without being swayed to give up.

BRAIN DRAIN

Everyone is losing so quickly; let me try to do what they're doing—only as a temporary measure!
Or,
I am losing so slowly that it's not even worth it.
I may as well enjoy it because I'm fat anyway.

BRAIN RETRAIN

There will always be a new quick fix, and there will always be a voice telling me to give up, but I will stay the course. Grit and consistency always win.

43
THE FOUR TENDENCIES

IN A PREVIOUS CHAPTER, we discussed bribing ourselves to stick to our commitments. Full disclosure: this doesn't work for everybody. If you are more internally motivated, external factors may have less sway over you than over those who are externally motivated.

There's a great book on different personality profiles, called *The Four Tendencies*, by Gretchen Rubin. In her book, she categorizes people as having one of four different tendencies that inform how they stay motivated. These include responding to inner expectations, outer expectations, both, or neither.

Her Four Tendencies are as follows:

The Upholder: Responds readily to both inner and outer expectations. Upholders thrive on meeting expectations, whether it's a deadline they set for themselves, or a task assigned by someone else.

The Questioner: Questions all expectations, only meeting them if those expectations make sense to them. Questioners need to understand the reasoning behind any expectation before they'll commit to it.

The Obliger: Meets outer expectations but struggles with inner expectations. Obligers have no problem keeping promises to others, but struggle when it comes to making time for their own goals.

The Rebel: Resists all expectations, outer and inner alike. Rebels resist control and often do the opposite of what they're told, even if it's something they want to do.

Understanding your tendency will give you a framework for what helps you stick to your plan because, at the end of the day, the challenge isn't to come up with the plan; the challenge is to adhere to the plan.

Adherence is the primary driver of results, especially when it comes to health and weight loss.

Let's go through each "Tendency" individually, and get to know the weaknesses, strengths, and suggested strategies for each profile.

THE UPHOLDER

The Upholder meets both inner and outer expectations.

For the select few of my clients, literally any plan or structure works. These are my Upholders. These clients really just need help creating a realistic plan and a bit of follow-up, but once they have that, they are good to go. Their intrinsic motivation is so powerful and their response to outer expectations is so strong, that they can accomplish amazing feats apparently all on their own, with just a little guidance.

The strength of the Upholder is their independence, and their belief that they can achieve their goals. Upholders are also very good at sticking to a plan exactly as written and perfectly following instructions, which is also a recipe for good results. The weakness of the Upholder is that they may end up being the perfectionists that we spoke about in chapter 27. When faced with challenges, they are prone to falling into black-and-white thinking patterns that lead to discouragement. If you believe that you are an Upholder, refer to chapter 27.

THE QUESTIONER

The Questioner meets inner expectations but resists outer ones.

Questioners are the least likely to find bribery effective. For the Questioner to successfully stay on plan, the plan needs to (1) make sense to them, (2) be fundamentally in alignment with their principles and intuition, and (3) be sufficiently flexible that they can control it and modify it themselves.

A Questioner may present like an Upholder, in terms of being an independent thinker. The main difference is that Upholders are fantastic at following instructions down to the tiniest detail, while Questioners are less perfectionistic in nature and may take liberties with small adjustments and tweaks. These small changes and liberties can end up being the very details that derail their success. If you are a Questioner, my advice would be to push yourself to stick to the details of the plan. Pick something, stick with it, and make the modifications you need, but remember that adherence is key.

THE OBLIGER

The Obliger meets outer expectations but resists inner expectations.

The Obliger is the most common of the Four Tendencies, which is why the bribery technique got its own chapter. Obligers are people-pleasers in the sense that they are more likely to do something when someone else expects it of them than for themselves. They tend to require more support and encouragement than the Upholders and will not stick to a plan or make progress independently, because they do not respond to their own internal motivation.

Obligers need workout buddies, personal trainers, nutrition coaches, and other external motivators. They need someone to hold them accountable in real time. Their strength is that once they have the slight pressure of an external source of expectation, most Obligers do a fantastic job of staying on track.

The weaknesses of the Obliger are vacations, business trips, and family pressure—in other words, any time the external pressure to exercise or eat well is removed or replaced by a less positive influence. My Obliger clients often experience setbacks on *Shabbosim*, *Yamim Tovim*, or trips, because they lack an internal compass of self-powered adherence. They are also more likely to give in to social pressure to overeat.

THE REBEL

The Rebel resists both inner and outer expectations.

Rebels often present as Obligers—they are discouraged, have "tried everything," never see results, and come in because they know they need help. However, the difference between Rebels and Obligers is that Obligers will follow a nutrition plan pretty accurately if you support them, while a Rebel will inexplicably fall off the wagon, even with your support. They tend to self-sabotage and come up with all the reasons why they can't lose weight. Somehow, they feel that they alone are different and that conventional ideas won't work for them.

If you think you may be a Rebel, your path may indeed be unconventional—not because you are truly different—but because motivation is all about adherence, and Rebels, by nature, have trouble with adherence. If you are a Rebel, you need to find a path that works for you.

To all the Rebels out there, here is my advice: Find something you love and that makes you feel good, and don't let other people pressure you. Be your unique, creative, and unorthodox self in the world of fitness and health, and you will be an inspiration to other Rebels around you.

BRAIN DRAIN

I have done plenty of diets in the past, but I am not sure I know how to stay on any plan long term.

BRAIN RETRAIN

Adherence is key. By identifying my personality profile, I will be more prepared for the long haul.

44
WHAT ABOUT EXERCISE?

YOU MAY HAVE noticed that I haven't talked much about exercise at all. In fact, if you do a search, you'll notice that this is pretty much my first mention of it. Okay, so let's talk about exercise. The reason I haven't brought it up until now is simple. Our body weight is 90 percent determined based on our food intake. That's right. You can pretty much reach and maintain your goal weight without ever exercising. And the opposite is true as well. You can exercise relentlessly, but if you have poor eating habits, you may never reach your weight loss goals.

Why? A few reasons. First of all, people tend to overestimate how many calories they burn during exercise and tend to make up for it either consciously or subconsciously by eating more. We may consciously justify some extra calories as long as we make sure that the extra calorie intake is lower than the calories expended through exercise. And we may subconsciously end up eating more because the exercise caused us to be hungrier than usual.

Second, while in the long term, exercise can turn us into energy-burning machines, allowing us to eat more without gaining weight, in the short term, we can actually gain a few pounds. This gain is caused by short-term inflammation (what we call "charley horse") and from muscle gain, as muscle weighs more than fat. While weighing more doesn't actually mean looking larger, and in fact, when taking measurements, the inches are clearly reducing, watching the scale go up can be aggravating.

I can't tell you how many times I have heard clients say, "I am following my food plan and exercising, and the scale won't budge," to which I tell them, "Okay, so stop exercising." And I mean it. At least temporarily, it might be better for them to see their hard work pay off on the scale by losing weight through their food plan. Once the weight is off, they can pick up where they left off with the exercise. As I always tell my clients, there is no emergency here. If it feels like too much work to exercise and diet, first get thin and then get fit. It is also much more rewarding to actually be able to see your muscles becoming more defined without that extra layer of fat blocking your view.

This is not to say that I don't believe in exercise. Exercise is critical for your health, mood, longevity, and weight control. But if you find that it is derailing your progress, whether physically or emotionally, it doesn't hurt to cool it off for a bit. This isn't a public service announcement for a lazy or sedentary lifestyle. We can and should be able to build activity and movement into our day without any of the possible negative effects listed above. This is simply a caution against potential burnout and frustration.

Here's a quick little pros and cons chart about exercising:

PROS

- Improves your overall health and wellness.
- Improves your mood.
- Burns calories.
- Builds muscle over time, which will boost your daily calorie burn and metabolism.
- May allow you to stay on plan because you won't want to "mess up" all your hard work.

CONS

- We tend to overestimate how many calories we burned and may be inclined to eat more because we burned so many calories. (PSA: Your treadmill is probably overestimating your calorie burn as well.) This can subconsciously give us permission to overeat.

- You may get very hungry from vigorous exercise and find it harder to stick to your food plan.
- If you are inflamed or charley horse from your workout, you may see the scale move higher, which can be emotionally frustrating, leading you to believe that your weight is stuck and that you can't lose.
- Muscle is heavier than fat, and therefore, you may end up weighing more, which can be frustrating for some people.
- If you are very overweight and/or don't enjoy exercising, you may feel that the weight loss process is very hard, when in truth, weight loss can be accomplished without exercise.

To exercise or not to exercise? This is your journey and, therefore, your choice. But the way I see it, if you already have an exercise routine that you enjoy, definitely continue what you are doing. If you aren't currently exercising and really don't want to start, hold off for a bit. Focus on your eating habits, lose some weight, and then see if you feel more motivated to begin.

Many of my clients get thin and only then get fit. And getting into exercising without the extra layers of body fat allows you to see more immediate progress. If you are ambivalent and don't have strong feelings either way, I would recommend moderate exercise. Find something that you enjoy and can commit to regularly, but don't overdo it. This way you can avoid most of the cons listed above while still reaping the benefits of the pros.

BRAIN DRAIN

I can eat what I want as long as I exercise.

BRAIN RETRAIN

Exercise is vital for my health and well-being. Watching what I eat is the key to maintaining my weight.

45

I THINK I HIT A PLATEAU...NOW WHAT?

ONE OF THE MOST frustrating experiences for dieters is hitting a plateau. The good news is that (1) a plateau is a good thing, not a bad thing, and (2) you probably haven't hit one yet.

Well, you might have, but first we need to make sure that the food isn't the problem.

When we start a new weight loss program, we are usually good little soldiers, doing everything right, and flying high on the wings of success. As we go on with our day-to-day lives, it's very possible that some of our old habits will creep back in without us realizing it. Double-check and make sure that you are still preparing your food, eating on schedule, and sticking to your recommended portion sizes. Make sure that little nibbles and extra bites aren't finding their way in. PSA: If you even out the cake while standing, the calories still count.

Very often, Shabbos is the culprit. Or our attitude toward it. Many people are great at staying disciplined during the week, when they are in their normal work routine, but they let loose a bit over Shabbos—*neshamah yeseirah* and all that good stuff. A good way to test if this is the case, aside from tracking our food, is the Shabbos scale test.

Step 1: Weigh yourself on Monday morning and write it down. Let's call this Weight A.

Step 2: Weigh yourself again on Friday morning, before Shabbos, and write down that weight as well. We will call this Weight B.

Step 3: Then weigh yourself the following Monday (exactly a week from the first time) and write it down. This will be called Weight C.

Now, let's analyze.

If your Friday weight, Weight B, is lower than your Monday weight Weight A, that means that your weekday food plan is fine, and you don't need to cut any calories, because your body has not really reached a plateau.

If your Monday weight Weight C is higher than the Friday weight, Weight B, it means you are likely eating too much over Shabbos, and are, therefore, spending too many days undoing the gain from Shabbos. Your focus should be on shaving calories that are finding their way in over Shabbos, when things are less scheduled and meals are bigger.

If, however, you didn't lose any weight from Monday to Friday, you are likely at a plateau, and congratulations are in order. In this case, please refer to the next chapter.

Aside from straying slightly from your plan, there are many reasons that your weight loss might have stalled even if you have been sticking to your plan, including the following:

- Travel—it can leave you constipated or bloated.
- Yom Tov—even if you did a great job with your food choices, the meals are often larger and later than usual.
- Hormonal fluctuations.
- Physical changes—lack of sleep, being sick, taking antibiotics.

It's very possible that you're experiencing a "Series of Unfortunate Events." This is the phenomenon whereby there are several weeks in a row that aren't conducive to weight loss for any of the above-mentioned reasons, which makes it seem like you have stopped losing weight, but, in actuality, you just haven't had the opportunity to lose.

For example, suppose you're a woman and you usually weigh yourself once a week on Friday mornings. If you weighed yourself one week while bloated from a dinner out, and then the following week your period was coming, and then the week after was right after a family vacation, you may go almost an entire month without seeing any weight loss. This doesn't mean you won't lose weight anymore. It just means that life is happening. This is not a true plateau.

One other factor to consider is exercise. If you have recently begun an exercise regimen, you may be building muscle, which weighs more than fat. This might make it seem like your weight loss has stalled, but you are likely still shedding fat and gaining muscle. If you believe this may be the case, you might want to do two things:

Take your measurements. By simply measuring your waist and hips once or twice a month, you will be able to see that while the pounds might not be dropping, the inches are.

Adjust your goal. If you were hoping to be 150 pounds, you may want to adjust that to be a muscular, toned 160 pounds.

If any of the above might be the case, try to practice patience. Remember that most people quit their diets because of frustration. Don't be one of those people. Stick to your plan, and the weight loss should pick back up when your body and routine go back to normal.

BRAIN DRAIN

My weight is stuck. This isn't working. I quit.

BRAIN RETRAIN

There are many reasons why my weight loss may have stalled. I will work toward identifying the problem and fixing it, rather than getting frustrated or using it as an excuse to quit.

46

CONGRATULATIONS! YOU HAVE HIT A PLATEAU!

YOU MAY BE wondering what I am so excited about here, as most people see a weight loss plateau as something negative or a sign that something is wrong. Not at all.

If you weighed 190 pounds when you started your weight loss journey, and were aiming for a goal of 140 pounds, it is normal for weight loss to plateau at about 170 pounds. That is because, as we stated in the beginning of this book, dieting should never be dramatic, as the body will physiologically rebel and make every effort to gain weight back in order to go back to its comfortable state, also known as homeostasis.

Therefore, the weight loss plan that we created at the beginning of the book is specifically designed to allow you to lose incrementally. The goal is to lose approximately 10 percent of your body weight at a time, at which point you adjust your food plan slightly to lose the next 10 percent. This way there is no extreme dieting, no dramatic hunger, and no rebound effect. Back to our example, if you have lost about 10 percent of your body weight, and now find yourself weighing about 170 pounds, you have done everything right. Losing the next 10 percent is supposed to require some tweaking and adjusting.

The good news is that it won't take much to kick the weight loss back into gear. You need to simply find ways to cut about 150–200 calories per day from your current plan. This can be done in one of several ways.

If you haven't done so already, it is a good idea to review the plan you created for yourself and see if you have strayed from it in any significant way. It is normal to eat more than you originally planned, and for many people, once they see that they can get away with those extras and still lose weight, the extras pretty much become part of their plan. If you're grabbing a handful of nuts here and there or tasting a few spoons of dinner before you serve yourself or your family, these calories can add up. While I'm all for eating those extras if you can have them and still lose weight, identifying those extras and cutting them out can be the first step toward shaving a couple hundred calories off your food plan when a plateau hits.

In other words, go back to the basics and track every bite that you eat: you will probably find some sneaky calories that found their way in and can be removed pretty easily without you feeling too much extra hunger. In fact, once you hit a plateau, your food plan should feel pretty easy to stick to because there is no longer a significant calorie deficit.

If you can't find anywhere to clean up your act, the next step to busting the plateau would be to cut some food from your original plan. Choosing lower-calorie snacks or lower-calorie protein options, such as chicken breast or egg whites, can save you some calories. Skipping your starch at dinner a few times a week, or swapping it out for a starchy vegetable instead, can also help.

However, it is important to remember that we don't want to cut out any complete meals or snacks because this will leave a long gap in your day without food. Going too long without food isn't conducive to sustainable weight loss. By now, you know that skipping meals or snacks will have the effect of slowing your metabolism over time. It also leaves you overly hungry, which will likely cause you to eventually eat more, not less. If it is indeed time to cut, please cut with caution.

BRAIN DRAIN

I have officially hit a plateau. My weight is really stuck.

BRAIN RETRAIN

A plateau is a milestone. My body is smaller and requires less food now, and I'm ready to cut some calories in order to keep losing. Time to level up.

47

TIME TO CUT!

AS WE DISCUSSED in the previous chapter, when you hit a plateau, it is time to shave some food from your original food plan. You don't have to cut too many calories per day in order to jump-start your weight loss again; two hundred to three hundred calories (or possibly less) per day should do the trick.

Here are some easy swaps that you can make without skipping any meals or snacks and without depriving yourself.

INSTEAD OF THIS:	CALORIE COUNT	CHOOSE THIS:	CALORIE COUNT	CALORIES SAVED
Mayonnaise, 1 tbsp.	120 calories	Low-fat mayonnaise, 1 tbsp.	30 calories	90 calories
Whole wheat bagel	350 calories	Bagel thins	100 calories	250 calories
2 eggs + 1 tsp. butter	200 calories	1 egg + 2 egg whites + cooking spray	100 calories	100 calories
Craisins, ¼ cup	225 calories	Blueberries, 1 cup	85 calories	140 calories
Microwave popcorn (mini bag), 4 cups	250 calories	Air-popped popcorn, 4 cups	150 calories	100 calories

INSTEAD OF THIS:	CALORIE COUNT	CHOOSE THIS:	CALORIE COUNT	CALORIES SAVED
Ben and Jerry's ice cream, ½ cup	300 calories	Halo Top ice cream, ½ cup	75 calories	225 calories
Olive oil, 1 tbsp.	120 calories	Olive oil spray	0 calories	120 calories
Granola, ½ cup	250 calories	All-Bran cereal	75 calories	175 calories
Spaghetti, cooked, ½ cup	200 calories	Spiralized zoodles, 1½ cups	25 calories	175 calories
Tortilla chips, 1 oz.	150 calories	Sliced radishes, 1 cup	15 calories	135 calories
Low-fat vanilla yogurt	140 calories	Plain Greek yogurt	80 calories	60 calories
Low-fat milk, 1 cup	120 calories	Unsweet-ened almond milk, 1 cup	30 calories	90 calories
PowerBar Peanut Butter Energy Bar	250 calories	ThinkThin High-Protein Bar	150 calories	100 calories
Rib-eye steak, 6 oz.	380 calories	Strip steak, 6 oz.	300 calories	80 calories
Peanut butter, 2 tbsp.	180 calories	PB2 peanut butter powder, 2 tbsp.	50 calories	130 calories

INSTEAD OF THIS:	CALORIE COUNT	CHOOSE THIS:	CALORIE COUNT	CALORIES SAVED
Margarita	325 calories	Diet Sprite with 2 shots Tequila	120 calories	205 calories
Hickory Smoke BBQ sauce, 2 tbsp.	50 calories	Mustard, 2 tsp.	5 calories	45 calories
2 chicken drumsticks with skin	300 calories	4 oz. chicken breast	150 calories	150 calories
Cooked rice, ½ cup	150 calories	Riced cauliflower, 1 cup	50 calories	100 calories
Mango, 1 large	200 calories	Apricots, 5 fresh	100 calories	100 calories
Dates, 3 large	200 calories	Prunes, 3 large	100 calories	100 calories
Ground beef, 6 oz.	400 calories	Ground veal, 6 oz.	250 calories	150 calories

As you see, cutting a couple hundred calories per day can be almost effortless. Go through your food log from the past few weeks, and see where you can save some calories. If you can't find any way to save, you can also shave a few ounces off of your serving sizes, or temporarily reduce your treat allotment. If you truly can't find anywhere to cut from, you might want to consider that your body has reached its set point.

In other words, your body might be telling you that it has reached the lowest weight that it can go without drastic measures. Skipping meals or snacks may allow you to temporarily go below your body's set point, but it is not a long-term solution because it is not sustainable. But taking a good look at your food log and analyzing your choices should yield some wiggle room to cut back without deprivation or hunger.

> BRAIN DRAIN
> I will have to go hungry in order to break through this plateau.
>
> BRAIN RETRAIN
> Jump-starting my weight loss will take a bit of skill as well as some attention to detail, but it should not leave me feeling hungry or deprived.

48

IT'S NOT ALWAYS THE FOOD

IN MY PRACTICE, I have found that, at some point, people hit a wall. This is different from a plateau, which we discussed in the last chapter. Sometimes, a client will stop losing weight for reasons that are unrelated to food.

Here is a list of other factors that may have stalled your weight loss:

- Stress—more than the usual
- Vitamin D deficiency
- Thyroid disorders
- For women: hormonal changes (aside from the usual month-to-month fluctuations, intentionally skipping periods would fall into this category as well)
- Lack of sleep

If any of these might be factors in your life, please do your best to address them, as I have found these to be the five reasons that weight loss mysteriously comes to a standstill. Food isn't always the culprit.

Take a few minutes to evaluate whether any of the above can be impeding your weight loss and to make moves to address those issues. If your stress levels are particularly high or your sleep is poor, please address it with your doctor or therapist. If you suspect vitamin D deficiency either because of a family history or because you have been deficient in the past, don't wait for your next doctor's appointment—it doesn't hurt to go to the health food store and take some vitamin D. Hormonal changes and thyroid issues can be dealt with as well. But please, don't remain stuck—take action!

We also have to consider our genetics, or our body's set point. If your weight is within a normal BMI and you have factored in all of the above and ruled them all out, it is possible that you may have to accept that your body doesn't want to shed those last few pounds and is going to put up a really good fight. That is not to say that you can't lose those last few pounds, but ask yourself, At what cost? Will I have to starve in order to get there? And will I have to continue to starve in order to stay there? You may want to accept that those few pounds are not worth the battle.

BRAIN DRAIN

My body just doesn't want to go any lower no matter what I do.

BRAIN RETRAIN

There are many factors that affect weight loss, and I'll address them all before making assumptions about my body.

49

THE DELICATE ART OF MAINTENANCE

YOU DID IT! You reached your goal weight. Whether this took you six weeks, six months, or a year (or more), congratulations are in order. It takes a tremendous amount of discipline to reach your goal weight, and you may have noticed that, as time went on, sticking to your food plan got more difficult rather than less so. Allow me to share a letter that I received a short while ago, and my response, which was published as part of a health column that I authored.

Dear Basya,

I set a goal three months ago to lose twenty pounds, and two weeks ago I reached my goal! I was so thrilled with how easily the weight came off. I never felt hungry, and I really enjoyed my food plan. However, since reaching my goal weight, I have really been struggling. I find myself eating foods I hadn't planned on eating and nibbling little extras here and there. I have already gained back two pounds, and I am so disappointed. What is going on? Where has my self-control gone? Please advise!

Signed,

Frustrated with maintenance

Dear Frustrated,

You are not alone! For so many dieters, losing is the fun part, and maintenance is the hard part. Losing a pound or two a week is a thrill. The fruits of your labor show up each week on the scale, and this motivates you to continue your hard work. Maintenance, on the other hand, is still a lot of work, but it almost feels like it's for nothing—the best-case scenario is that the scale stays the same—none of that thrill of losing.

Also, when someone has twenty pounds to lose (or thirty or fifty), there is a level of desperation that drives most people to stay on track. It is as if they hit rock bottom, and their determination to lose is stronger than any temptation. As maintenance nears, that desperation is gone. Of course, there is a desire not to gain weight back, but it has a lesser intensity to it than the determination to lose the extra weight.

The key to successful maintenance is to realize that maintenance is hard work. If you saw your diet as a temporary measure in order to drop the extra weight, the time to shift that mentality is now. Going back to your old habits will bring you slowly but steadily back to your old weight. Maintenance should look exactly like dieting, but with a controlled, moderate amount of extra food—foods you missed while you were dieting, or just larger portions worked in to keep you from either losing or gaining.

All the good habits that you developed while you were dieting should be incorporated permanently. This means tracking your food on a food log, preparing your food the night before, especially if you will be on the go the next day, weighing and measuring your food, sticking to a food schedule and routine, drinking your full amount of water, etc. Don't let go of these habits! They are just as important during maintenance as they were during the weight loss stage, if not more so. Also, remember how important it is to have accountability and support.

Finally, make sure to enjoy your maintenance. Buy new clothes. Take professional pictures. Savor the added food that you are allotting yourself on your maintenance plan. Be proud of your success. You worked hard for this weight loss; now go ahead and enjoy it.

Best wishes for continued success,

Basya Kovacs

I believe this says it all. If you have developed good habits over the course of the year, you are already ahead of the game. You have pushed through and persevered even when it was tough, and if you continue pushing, these habits will become second nature. But you need to keep fighting. New habits take time to develop, and many of the challenges you faced during the year only came up a handful of times. While the day-to-day routine may be easy by now, the exceptions to the rule such as Shabbos, Yom Tov, *simchas*, vacations, and other events may still be new. Keep on pushing because practice makes progress!

So, you're wondering how maintenance is any different from weight loss. It is different, but only slightly so. You still need all the skills and tools we discussed in this book. The only thing that really changes is how much food you eat. Instead of eating to lose weight, you will now be eating to maintain your weight. This will allow you a bit of wiggle room, likely two hundred to three hundred calories extra per day.

If you have reached your goal weight and would like to transition to a maintenance plan, here's the plan:

- Test out adding a few hundred calories to your food plan and see what happens. If you still lose weight after a week or two, you can add an additional few hundred calories. If you gain weight, it means you likely added too many calories, and will need to pull back. Play around with the calories until you find your happy place, where you are neither gaining nor losing.
- Your maintenance calories shouldn't be haphazard—randomness is not a plan. Grazing and nibbling and overindulging at random will make you feel out of control and will eventually lead to weight gain. Decide upon which extras you would like to incorporate, either at the beginning of each week or at the beginning of each day, and stick to it. For example, a half a bagel

or a chocolate bar, planned in the morning, can be a fun addition to your regular routine.

- While on maintenance it is still wise to continue to avoid foods that trigger you. If you know that once you start eating granola or white bread you can't stop, don't start.
- Continue weighing yourself once a week to make sure your weight isn't creeping up. If it is, just go back to your weight loss plan.

But most importantly, keep the rest of your skill set intact. Prep your food, keep your food log, eat on schedule, and make sure you have accountability. Use your skills and continue to develop your habits. Like the old saying goes—use it or lose it! Or in this case, use it or gain it!

BRAIN DRAIN

I did it! I reached my goal weight! Now I am free to eat as I please.

BRAIN RETRAIN

Maintenance is a milestone, and now I get to enjoy some extras. However, if I go back to my old eating habits, I will ultimately go back to my old weight. Maintenance is the next challenge—the beginning of forever—and I am ready!

50

WHY CAN'T I JUST BE NORMAL?

LET ME TELL YOU about two of my clients and their weight loss journeys. They have two very different dieting profiles but share a common sentiment that I believe we can all relate to.

The first woman, let's call her Miriam, has been a client for over two years. Petite and in her early fifties, Miriam successfully and quite easily lost over twenty-five pounds, but struggles mightily day after day to keep the weight off. The constant battle exhausts and frustrates her. At her most recent weigh-in, Miriam cried to me, "Am I really going to always have to be that crazy woman who brings her own healthy snacks wherever she goes? Do I really have to live this way forever?"

The second client, a recent college graduate, expressed a similar sentiment. This girl, let's call her Sarah, lost weight with a different nutritionist, on a very strictly regimented diet that cut out all snacks, sweets, treats, meats, and fun food. Of course, this type of plan is unsustainable, and her weight began to creep back on. Sarah came to me in order to try to maintain her weight loss while reintroducing all the foods she'd deprived herself of for many months. Session after session, burned out from her previous diet, Sarah kept telling me, "I just want to do whatever I want, and be normal!"

Both of these clients, and many others, are just yearning to be free from the burden of "dieting." Many of us feel the same way. We wish we could just eat when we were hungry and stop when we were full and live thinly ever after. If only it were this simple. If only we could be "free" and "normal."

Unfortunately, our version of "normal" is clouded by a host of factors, including but not limited to the following:

- We live busy lives and don't always know when we are hungry until we are well past the point of normal hunger.
- We are blessed with an (over)abundance of food in every grocery, pantry, and refrigerator beckoning to us at all times.
- Advertisements in magazines, media, blogs, and newspapers constantly bombard us to eat.
- An entire foodie culture encourages us to eat more, focus on food more, eat creatively, and eat constantly.
- Chemically engineered food is designed to keep us coming back for more. For example, high fructose corn syrup, MSG, and hydrogenated fats are intentionally added to make food as addictive as possible.

With all these factors at play, we can no longer trust our judgment or even our appetite. Being free to do whatever we want sounds lovely, until we realize that our wants and desires are swayed and manipulated by the forces at play as described above. The only way to truly enjoy all the different foods and all of life's occasions is to do so within a structure and a framework, also known as a diet.

Freedom, then, can't mean doing whatever we want when we want—because what we want is subject to change on a whim. Structure and rules are needed. Too many rules can suppress and suffocate us, but the right structure and framework actually sets us free!

So, yes, Miriam might need to bring her own healthy snacks when she goes away for Shabbos, because without them, she goes off track. And, yes, Sarah might never be able to just eat as much as she wants whenever she wants, because her appetite is larger than her caloric needs. But who is to say that others are more free? Is eating to your heart's content and then being filled with guilt and regret truly freedom? Is starving all day because you are too busy to eat, and then eating all night while feeling depressed and out of control true freedom? Having a structured framework that is consistent allows us to enjoy all foods in moderation, while remaining healthy and having the figure we want. This is true freedom.

BRAIN DRAIN

Why can't I just eat when I am hungry and stop when I am full? I am sick of all this dieting.

BRAIN RETRAIN

It is unrealistic to maintain a healthy body weight if we rely solely on our appetites, because there are many factors that influence how much we want to eat. Having a structure, a food plan, a schedule, and most of all, discipline, allows us to have the best of all worlds.

51

STAY ON THE ROAD AND HIT THE DEER

MANY PEOPLE HAVE a mistaken belief that once they lose their weight, they are somehow done. They believe that they did the work for three months, or six months or a year, and now they are entitled to reap the fruits of their labor for the rest of their lives. This is unfortunate, because if you go back to the way you used to eat, you will go back to the weight you used to weigh. It's very simple. The eating habits that caused you to become overweight will again cause you to become overweight, and the eating habits that allowed you to lose the weight are the same ones that will allow you to keep the weight off.

Because the weight creeps back up slowly, many people don't realize this basic concept right away. But if you find yourself gaining even half a pound a week, please realize that this will lead to a twenty-four-pound weight gain during the course of a year.

Please don't fool yourself into thinking that now that you have lost your extra weight, you are somehow exempt from the struggle that plagues almost 90 percent of American adults—"the battle of the bulge." Please keep fighting the good fight and stay in the game. The challenges will keep on coming, and we need to be prepared to keep on fighting.

Did you know that most fatal accidents involving deer on the road actually have nothing to do with hitting the deer? Now, I'm not underestimating how terrifying it is when you see that deer dart out in front of the car. That moment when both you and the deer look like a deer caught in the headlights isn't easily forgotten. But the real issue isn't actually hitting the deer. The deadly part of this scenario is when you panic, swerve desperately to avoid hitting the deer, and lose control of the car. That's how fatalities occur.

I remember when I took driver's ed, they taught us that if a deer gets in your way while driving, slow down, remain in control, brake calmly, and if it means that you hit the deer, hit the deer.

Why is all this relevant? Good question. When we go off plan, we may be caught off guard. We usually start out innocently. "A little bit won't hurt," or, "It's just a taste, just a bite, just the kids' leftovers." In other words, we believe the situation is still fixable. While not ideal, at least we are still conscious, and still in control. We can stop at any time. So far, all good.

But sometimes, when it goes too far, when we feel like we really messed up, the tune changes. Then we start to say things like, "I'll get back on track after Shabbos, or after Yom Tov, or after my next weigh-in with my nutritionist." This is when the real trouble starts, because now, we are basically saying, "I give up," and with relief, we kick it down the line to worry about at a later date. Now, we can freely indulge without the stress of justifying each bite. Uh-oh. Suddenly, we are swerving wildly out of control.

What a mistake. Once we do this, we have permission to derail without worrying about it for the next few days or weeks, until the random deadline we made to soothe ourselves. And by the time we brush ourselves off, we often have several extra pounds to deal with. Had we stayed present and in control, we could have avoided this entire scenario and stopped before too much damage was done.

Back to hitting the deer—this isn't so much about maiming animals as it is about the importance of remaining present and in control even if there's some damage. If I have to choose between hitting the deer and losing control, I say stay in control. The flip side is a car flipped over on the side of the road.

What does "staying on the road" look like?

Track your food in a food diary. Even if it's a mess of a tracking sheet, just keep writing it down. The act of writing forces you to stay present and somewhat in control.

Accountability. Make sure you answer to someone other than yourself. Don't avoid this part or push it off, no matter how disastrous your day or week was.

Learn from your mistakes. Figure out what went wrong and how to avoid it the next time.

This is pretty much it. These are the basics. If you are doing this, you are in control and you will rebound quickly, even if you mess up. As the saying goes—it doesn't get easier; you just get stronger. Just hit the deer, check your car for damage, and keep on driving.

BRAIN DRAIN

I give up—dieting is too hard, and I have failed too many times. I don't think I will get it right, so I may as well quit.

BRAIN RETRAIN

I just need to keep driving—I need to keep on learning from my mistakes and practicing my new thought processes. Derailing completely just prolongs the damage.

52
EYE ON THE PRIZE

WHEN A CLIENT struggles, I usually offer that he or she check in with me on a nightly basis. By reaching out and sending a daily food log, we are offering a higher level of support and accountability, which usually helps the client get back into a good routine. While this does take a bit of my time, I am happy to offer clients this option when I feel it will help. If my client is willing to go the extra mile by checking in nightly, I am willing to dedicate my time as well. I have seen amazing results with this extra level of accountability and support.

At times, I will have a client who, despite all my best efforts to help, will still struggle. Often, she will come into my office and say, "Basya, I need you to motivate me. I don't know what happened, but I just can't get hold of myself. At the beginning, I was so determined to lose weight, but I can't seem to get myself back into it—please inspire me!"

My response is usually some version of the following (spoiler alert: this might sound like a bit of tough love). I tell my client, "I could definitely inspire you—in fact, I consider myself a pretty motivational coach. But it won't help. Meaning, my acting as your motivational cheerleader will be effective until you walk out the door, or maybe until tomorrow. But then it will, once again, be gone." In other words, you need to find the motivation within yourself.

I try to remind my client that the weight loss process can at times be exciting, but more often than not, choosing to eat healthfully and moderately takes work. Of course, we try to make things easier by providing helpful ideas and troubleshooting tips, and by offering delicious snacks, treats, recipes of the week, and daily doses of inspiration, but at the end of the day, the change in lifestyle requires some discipline and sacrifice that may or may not be fun.

I like to use parenting as an example. When our children are acting sweet and getting along and not whining or complaining, we are super motivated to be good parents. But when the child becomes unreasonable and cranky, we need to do our job as nurturing parents despite the fact that it is suddenly an extreme test of our patience. When something is important enough, we need to do it despite it being difficult, whether we are motivated or not.

The bottom line is that just like anything worthwhile, we need to stick to it even when we aren't inspired. We need to be able to envision that the short-term sacrifice will lead to a long-term pleasure. In our weak moments, we need to remember that we are giving up instant gratification for a greater goal. The trick is to remember these goals in the moment of struggle. When we are feeling unmotivated and off-track, we need to be able to remind ourselves why we are even sacrificing.

When I tell my client that I can't motivate her, it's because the motivation can't come from me. I try to help my clients find the motivation within themselves. I try to help them access that same motivation that brought them into my office in the first place, because only that kind of motivation has the long-term power needed to lose the weight and keep it off.

Remember at the beginning of this book I suggested that you "find your why." You wrote down all the reasons that you wanted to lose weight. You had a clear picture of what you would get out of this—why all this hard work was worth it. Reread that list daily. Even twice a day. Remind yourself why this is so important to you. This way when you feel frustrated or ready to throw in the towel, this list will be readily accessible.

Not too long ago, one of my twins came home from school seeming really upset. When I asked him what was bothering him, he told me with tears running down his face, "Aron asked me for my snack, and I gave it to him, and then I didn't have any snack. I didn't want to give it to him! I wanted it for myself!" After a few minutes of me empathizing with him about how rough it must have been to have no snack, he recovered, and went on with his evening.

I, on the other hand, was left pondering. Eli wanted his snack. Snacks are important and delicious. But he also wanted his friendship with Aron. Aron isn't a bully, and didn't make him give him the snack. He requested it, and my son decided to share. I realized that though it didn't look like it on the surface, Eli had been faced with two good options: (1) keep and enjoy his bag of chips or (2) strengthen his relationship with a friend, or at the very least, not put it at risk. And I realized that my son made a choice, and even though it didn't feel like it, he did exactly as he wanted.

The more I thought about it, the more I realized that most of the time we really do exactly as we want, even if it doesn't seem that way. For example, if someone feels forced to visit a friend even though she really isn't in the mood, and goes anyway, it might just mean that she values seeing herself (or having others see her) as a generous, kind person more than she values her free time. Or, if someone complies with family or social rules even if he doesn't have the same value system, that may mean that he values being accepted by a larger group more than he values his independence. In other words, even though we sometimes resent our own choices, we really do exactly what we want.

Of course, this made me think about sticking to a food plan. It made me realize that every time we are faced with temptation, we are given two good options, and whatever we choose reflects what we really want. When I tell my sisters and sisters-in-law that I don't want cake at a family gathering, it actually is the truth. I am well aware that cake is delicious, but I don't want it as strongly as I want to maintain my weight.

But we can only choose what we truly want when we are clear about our choices. Meaning, if I am at a party and I am choosing between having the cheesecake and not having the cheesecake, having the cheesecake definitely wins. Of course, I prefer cheesecake over no cheesecake. I am sane, after all. However, if my higher goal or value is clear in my mind, it is a completely different battle. It becomes the choice between having cheesecake and maintaining my weight! In this case, the choice is clear, and I am able to easily choose what is more valuable to me. I can make this decision more easily, and without resentment.

The key is keeping your weight loss and health goals clear and focused, front and center. This way, when faced with a food-related temptation, you are able to choose what you truly value more. And I'm willing to bet that it's your health and wellness, not the cheesecake.

BRAIN DRAIN

I am sacrificing so much and working so hard to maintain my weight.

BRAIN RETRAIN

My goals are crystal clear, and the choices I make toward those goals are not a sacrifice.

APPENDIX I

THE CYCLES OF FRUSTRATION AND THE CYCLE OF SUCCESS

IN MY YEARS as a coach, I have found some patterns that are almost universal. The most common of those patterns is the cycle of frustration in which people find themselves when they start their day with a very late breakfast. The second most common is similar, but it also includes what happens when people skip their meals or snacks. Both end in slowed weight loss and frustration.

The good news is that when the cycle is reversed (which I will admit can be challenging—we are busy people!) the results are also reversed.

The images on the following two pages depict the two most common cycles of frustration. If they seem at all familiar to you, you're sure to benefit from the image that follows after that!

CYCLES OF FRUSTRATION

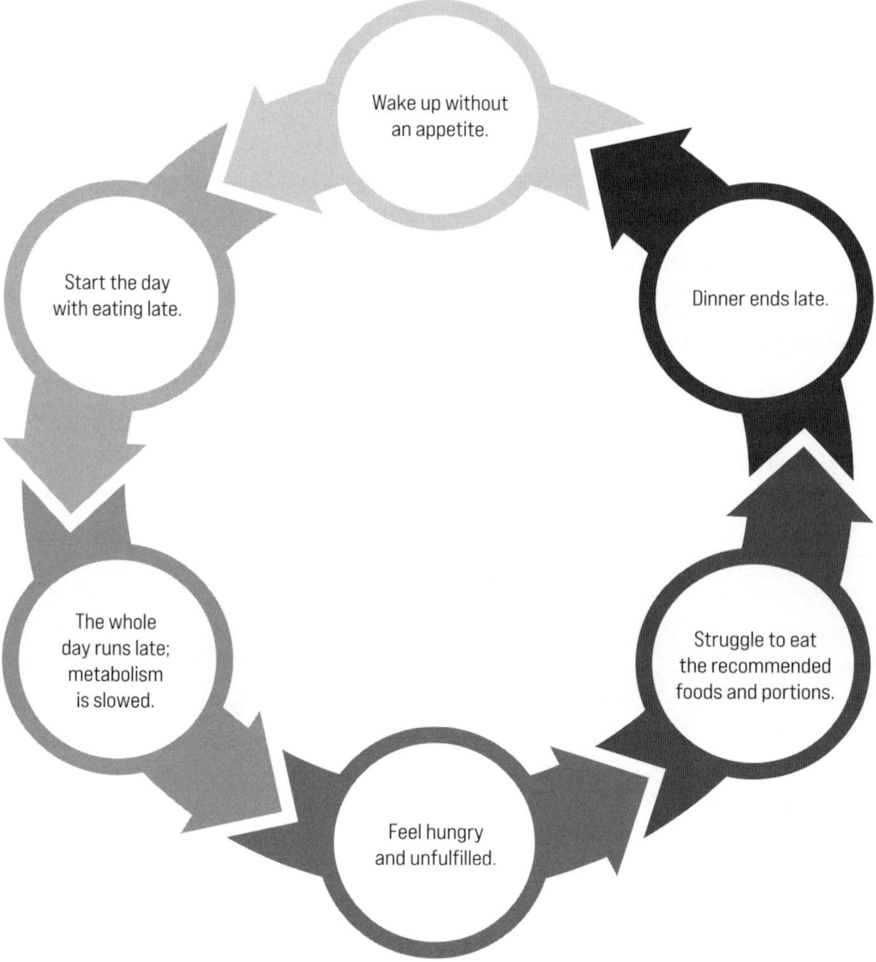

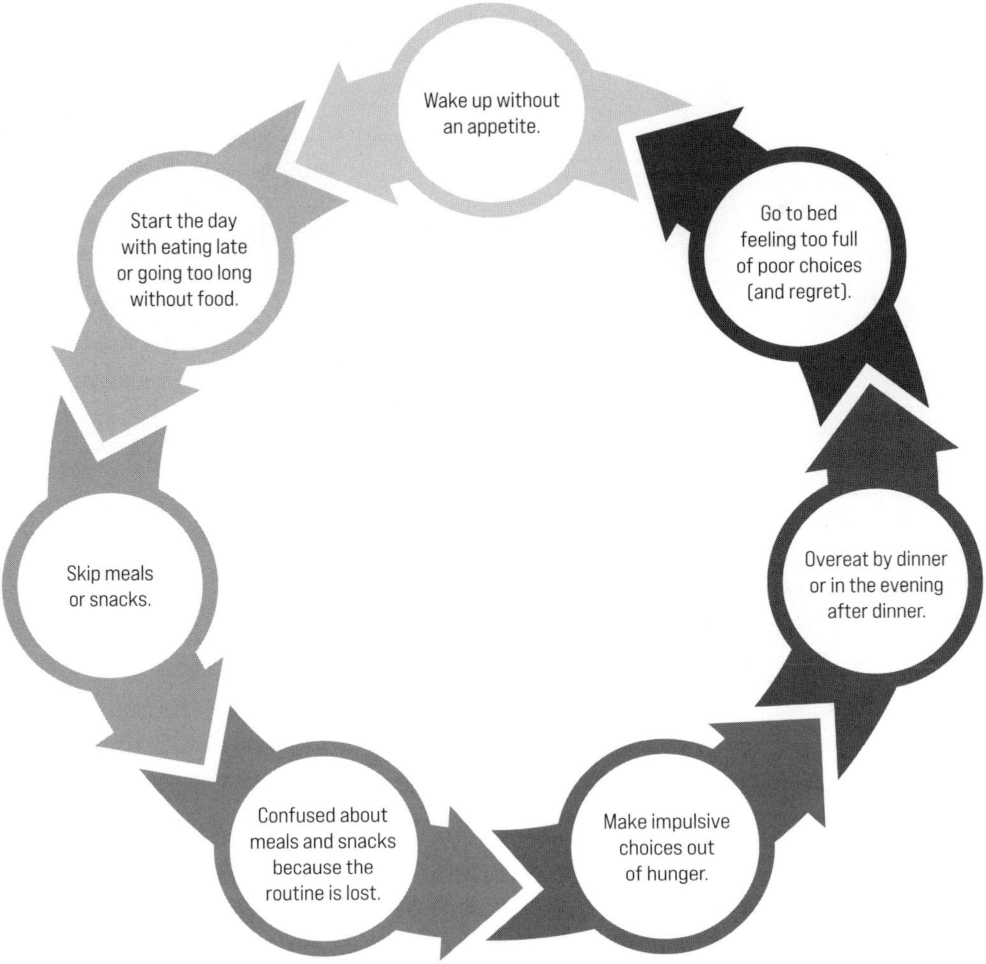
Wake up without an appetite.
Start the day with eating late or going too long without food.
Skip meals or snacks.
Confused about meals and snacks because the routine is lost.
Make impulsive choices out of hunger.
Overeat by dinner or in the evening after dinner.
Go to bed feeling too full of poor choices (and regret).

CYCLE OF SUCCESS

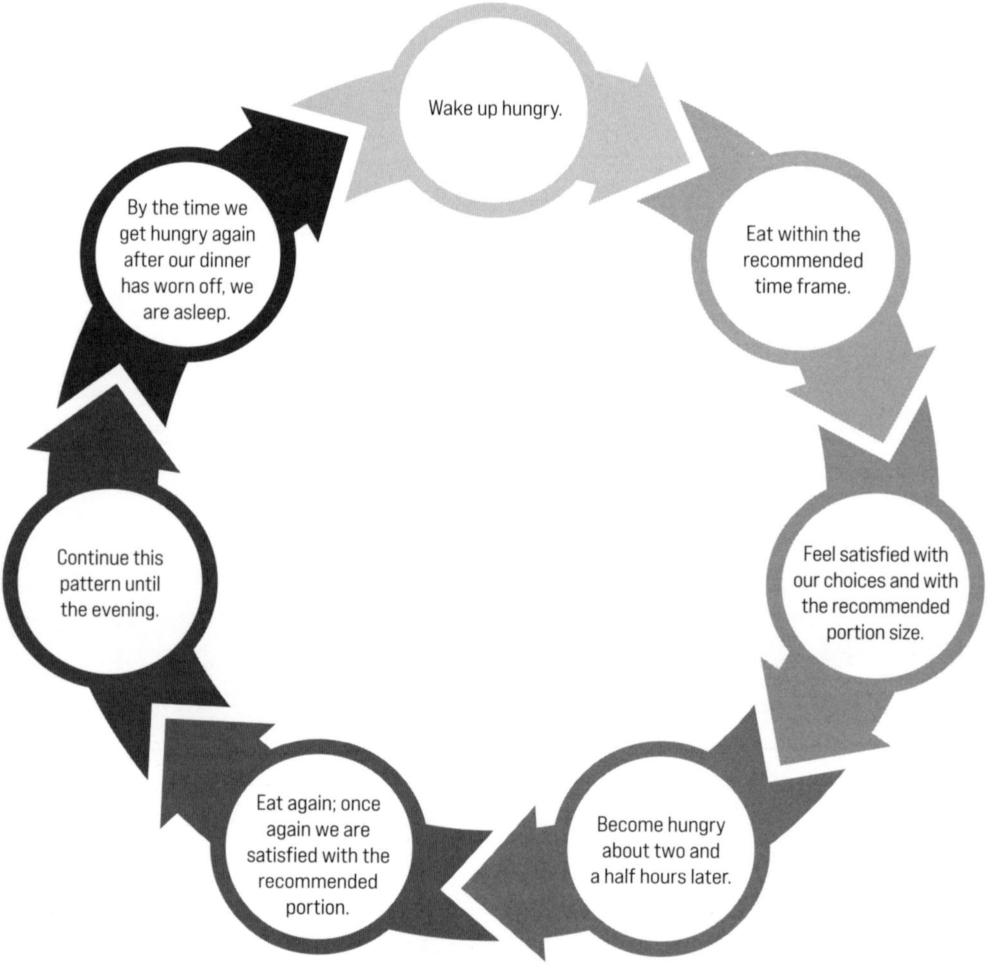

APPENDIX II

TORAH SOURCES ON EATING PROPERLY

Source Sheet by Yehuda Kovacs

THE TORAH is our guide, and all the wisdom of the world can be found in the Torah. The sources cited below make the following three key points:

1. Being overly restrictive in areas that are permitted is frowned upon by the Torah.
2. The cause of almost all illnesses is overeating (even healthy food!). Conversely, eating too little is also not healthy.
3. Food should be a source of both sustenance and pleasure, but eating should generally take place when one is in a good mood—not while stressed, worried, or angry.

משנה תורה, הלכות דעות א׳:ג׳

(ג) שְׁתֵּי קְצָווֹת הָרְחוֹקוֹת זוֹ מִזּוֹ שֶׁבְּכָל דֵּעָה וְדֵעָה אֵינָן דֶּרֶךְ טוֹבָה וְאֵין רָאוּי לוֹ לְאָדָם לָלֶכֶת בָּהֶן וְלֹא לְלַמְּדָן לְעַצְמוֹ. וְאִם מָצָא טִבְעוֹ נוֹטֶה לְאַחַת מֵהֶן אוֹ מוּכָן לְאַחַת מֵהֶן אוֹ שֶׁכְּבָר לָמֵד אַחַת מֵהֶן וְנָהַג בָּהּ יַחֲזִיר עַצְמוֹ לַמּוּטָב וְיֵלֵךְ בְּדֶרֶךְ הַטּוֹבִים וְהִיא הַדֶּרֶךְ הַיְשָׁרָה:

MISHNEH TORAH, HUMAN DISPOSITIONS 1:3

(3) The two extremes of each trait, which are at a distance from one another, do not reflect a proper path. It is not fitting that a man should behave in accordance with these extremes or teach them to himself.

If he finds that his nature leans toward one of the extremes or adapts itself easily to it, or if he has learned one of the extremes and acts accordingly, he should bring himself back to what is proper and walk in the path of the good [men]. This is the straight path.

משנה תורה, הלכות דעות ג׳:א׳

(א) שֶׁמָּא יֹאמַר אָדָם הוֹאִיל וְהַקִּנְאָה וְהַתַּאֲוָה וְהַכָּבוֹד וְכַיּוֹצֵא בָּהֶם דֶּרֶךְ רָעָה הֵן וּמוֹצִיאִין אֶת הָאָדָם מִן הָעוֹלָם. אֶפְרשׁ מֵהֶן בְּיוֹתֵר וְאֶתְרַחֵק לַצַּד הָאַחֲרוֹן. עַד שֶׁלֹּא יֹאכַל בָּשָׂר וְלֹא יִשְׁתֶּה יַיִן וְלֹא יִשָּׂא אִשָּׁה וְלֹא יֵשֵׁב בְּדִירָה נָאָה וְלֹא יִלְבַּשׁ מַלְבּוּשׁ נָאֶה אֶלָּא הַשַּׂק וְהַצֶּמֶר הַקָּשֶׁה וְכַיּוֹצֵא בָּהֶן כְּגוֹן כֹּהֲנֵי הָעוֹבְדֵי כּוֹכָבִים. גַּם זֶה דֶּרֶךְ רָעָה הִיא וְאָסוּר לֵילֵךְ בָּהּ. הַמְהַלֵּךְ בְּדֶרֶךְ זוֹ נִקְרָא חוֹטֵא. שֶׁהֲרֵי הוּא אוֹמֵר בְּנָזִיר (במדבר ו יא) "וְכִפֶּר עָלָיו מֵאֲשֶׁר חָטָא עַל הַנָּפֶשׁ". אָמְרוּ חֲכָמִים וּמָה אִם נָזִיר שֶׁלֹּא פֵּרַשׁ אֶלָּא מִן הַיַּיִן צָרִיךְ כַּפָּרָה הַמּוֹנֵעַ עַצְמוֹ מִכָּל דָּבָר וְדָבָר עַל אַחַת כַּמָּה וְכַמָּה. לְפִיכָךְ צִוּוּ חֲכָמִים שֶׁלֹּא יִמְנַע אָדָם עַצְמוֹ אֶלָּא מִדְּבָרִים שֶׁמְּנָעַתּוּ הַתּוֹרָה בִּלְבַד. וְלֹא יְהֵא אוֹסֵר עַצְמוֹ בִּנְדָרִים וּבִשְׁבוּעוֹת עַל דְּבָרִים הַמֻּתָּרִים. כָּךְ אָמְרוּ חֲכָמִים לֹא דַּיֵּךְ מַה שֶּׁאָסְרָה תּוֹרָה אֶלָּא שֶׁאַתָּה אוֹסֵר עָלֶיךָ דְּבָרִים אֲחֵרִים. וּבִכְלָל הַזֶּה אֵלּוּ שֶׁמִּתְעַנִּין תָּמִיד אֵינָן בְּדֶרֶךְ טוֹבָה. וְאָסְרוּ חֲכָמִים שֶׁיְּהֵא אָדָם מְסַגֵּף עַצְמוֹ בְּתַעֲנִית. וְעַל כָּל הַדְּבָרִים הָאֵלּוּ וְכַיּוֹצֵא בָּהֶן צִוָּה שְׁלֹמֹה וְאָמַר (קהלת ז טז) "אַל תְּהִי צַדִּיק הַרְבֵּה וְאַל תִּתְחַכַּם יוֹתֵר לָמָּה תִּשּׁוֹמֵם":

MISHNEH TORAH, HUMAN DISPOSITIONS 3:1

(1) A person might say, "Since envy, desire, [the pursuit] of honor, and the like, are a wrong path and drive a person from the world, I shall separate from them to a very great degree and move away from them to the opposite extreme." For example, he will not eat meat, nor drink wine, nor live in a pleasant home, nor wear fine clothing, but, rather, [wear] sackcloth and coarse wool and the like—just as the pagan priests do.

This, too, is a bad path, and it is forbidden to walk upon it. Whoever follows this path is called a sinner [as implied by the Bamidbar 6:11] statement concerning a nazir: "And he [the Kohen] shall make an atonement for him, for his having sinned regarding [his] soul." Our Sages declared: If the nazir who abstained only from wine requires atonement, how much more so does one who abstains from everything.

Therefore, our Sages directed man to abstain only from those things which the Torah denies him, and not to forbid

himself permitted things by vows and oaths [of abstention]. *Thus, our Sages stated: Are not those things which the Torah has prohibited sufficient for you that you must forbid additional things to yourself?*

This general statement also refers to those who fast constantly. They are not following a good path, [for] our Sages have forbidden a man to mortify himself by fasting. Of all the above, and their like, Shlomo directed and said: "Do not be overly righteous and do not be overly clever; why make yourself desolate?" (Koheles 7:16).

משנה תורה, הלכות דעות ג׳:ב׳

(ב)...וְכֵן כְּשֶׁיֹּאכַל וְיִשְׁתֶּה וְיִבְעֹל לֹא יָשִׂים בְּלִבּוֹ לַעֲשׂוֹת דְּבָרִים הָאֵלּוּ כְּדֵי לֵהָנוֹת בִּלְבַד עַד שֶׁנִּמְצָא שֶׁאֵינוֹ אוֹכֵל וְשׁוֹתֶה אֶלָּא הַמָּתוֹק לַחֵךְ וְיִבְעֹל כְּדֵי לֵהָנוֹת, אֶלָּא יָשִׂים עַל לִבּוֹ שֶׁיֹּאכַל וְיִשְׁתֶּה כְּדֵי לְהַבְרוֹת גּוּפוֹ וְאֵיבָרָיו בִּלְבַד. לְפִיכָךְ לֹא יֹאכַל כָּל שֶׁהַחֵךְ מִתְאַוֶּה כְּכֶלֶב וַחֲמוֹר אֶלָּא יֹאכַל דְּבָרִים הַמּוֹעִילִים לַגּוּף אִם מָרִים אִם מְתוּקִים. וְלֹא יֹאכַל דְּבָרִים הָרָעִים לַגּוּף אַף עַל פִּי שֶׁהֵן מְתוּקִים לַחֵךְ. כֵּיצַד? מִי שֶׁהָיָה בְּשָׂרוֹ חַם לֹא יֹאכַל בָּשָׂר וְלֹא דְּבַשׁ וְלֹא יִשְׁתֶּה יַיִן, כְּעִנְיָן שֶׁאָמַר שְׁלֹמֹה דֶּרֶךְ מָשָׁל (משלי כה כז) "אָכֹל דְּבַשׁ" וְגוֹ׳. וְשׁוֹתֶה מֵי הָעֻלְשִׁין אַף עַל פִּי שֶׁהוּא מַר שֶׁנִּמְצָא שׁוֹתֶה וְאוֹכֵל דֶּרֶךְ רְפוּאָה בִּלְבַד כְּדֵי שֶׁיַּבְרִיא וְיַעֲמֹד שָׁלֵם הוֹאִיל וְאִי אֶפְשָׁר לָאָדָם לִחְיוֹת אֶלָּא בַּאֲכִילָה וּשְׁתִיָּה.

MISHNEH TORAH, HUMAN DISPOSITIONS 3:2

Similarly, when he eats, drinks, and engages in intimate relations, he should not intend to do these things solely for pleasure to the point where he will eat and drink only that which is sweet to the palate and engage in intercourse for pleasure. Rather, he should take care to eat and drink only in order to be healthy in body and limb.

Therefore, he should not eat all that the palate desires like a dog or a donkey. Rather, he should eat what is beneficial for the body, be it bitter or sweet. Conversely, he should not eat what is harmful to the body, even though it is sweet to the palate. For example: a person with a warm constitution should not eat meat or honey, nor drink wine, as Shlomo has stated in a parable: The eating of much honey is not good (Mishlei 25:27). One should drink endive juice, even though it is bitter, for then, ***he will be eating and drinking for medical reasons only, in order to become healthy and be whole—for a man cannot exist without eating and drinking.***

משנה תורה, הלכות דעות ד׳:ט״ו

וַאֲכִילָה גַּסָּה לְגוּף כָּל אָדָם כְּמוֹ סַם הַמָּוֶת. וְהוּא עִקָּר לְכָל הֶחֳלָאִים. וְרֹב הֶחֳלָאִים שֶׁבָּאִים עַל הָאָדָם אֵינָם אֶלָּא אוֹ מִפְּנֵי מַאֲכָלִים רָעִים. אוֹ מִפְּנֵי שֶׁהוּא מְמַלֵּא בִּטְנוֹ וְאוֹכֵל אֲכִילָה גַּסָּה אֲפִלּוּ מִמַּאֲכָלִים טוֹבִים. הוּא שֶׁשְּׁלֹמֹה אָמַר בְּחָכְמָתוֹ (משלי כא כג) "שֹׁמֵר פִּיו וּלְשׁוֹנוֹ שֹׁמֵר מִצָּרוֹת נַפְשׁוֹ". כְּלוֹמַר שׁוֹמֵר פִּיו מִלֶּאֱכֹל מַאֲכָל רַע אוֹ מִלִּשְׂבַּע וּלְשׁוֹנוֹ מִלְּדַבֵּר אֶלָּא בִּצְרָכָיו:

MISHNEH TORAH, HUMAN DISPOSITIONS 4:15

Overeating is like poison to anyone's body. It is the main source of all illness. ***Most illnesses which afflict a man are caused by harmful foods or by his filling his belly and overeating, even of healthful foods.***

This was implied by Shlomo in his wisdom: "Whoever guards his mouth and his tongue, guards his soul from distress" (Mishlei 21:23), i.e., "guards his mouth" from eating harmful food or eating his fill and "his tongue" from speaking [about things] other than his needs.

קיצור שלחן ערוך ל״ב:כ״ב

וּמִכָּל שֶׁכֵּן שֶׁצָּרִיךְ לִזָּהֵר שֶׁלֹּא יֹאכַל כְּשֶׁהוּא בְּכַעַס אוֹ בְּפַחַד אוֹ בִּדְאָגָה, אֶלָּא כְּשֶׁהוּא בְּשִׂמְחָה מְמֻצַּעַת.

KITZUR SHULCHAN ARUCH 32:22

Needless to say, you should be careful not to eat when angry, fearful, or anxious, but rather when in a moderately joyful mood.

P'SAK FROM RABBI YISROEL DERBAREMDIGER REGARDING BAL TASHCHIS

Greetings to your staff, who faithfully carry out their duties in training the public regarding healthy eating habits using the BKCoaching diet method.

You have requested that I write my opinion about a question that many of your clients ask—the prohibition of bal tashchis, i.e., discarding edible foods into the garbage. The question is whether it is permitted to throw out foods that are still good but are not healthy and are not useful for the client's diet.

In truth, the prohibition of destroying a useful item is (in the opinion of the majority Rishonim) a Torah prohibition.[1] *However, in this situation it is clear that it is permissible to throw them out and* ***it is even considered a mitzvah****. The Gemara in Shabbos 129a says that one is allowed to destroy vessels in order to save oneself from bodily harm. In the words of the Gemara, "Bal tashchis of the body is a higher priority." The reasoning behind this is as follows. The root of the prohibition is because the Torah wants us to use every creation to its ultimate benefit and not to cause destruction to any object. Behold, Yaakov Avinu even went back to retrieve small jugs! This, however, only applies when it is done in a manner of destruction and waste. If, however, by saving an item, it will harm a human being, who is the most important creature in the world, then certainly not causing physical harm is more important, and it is not even considered destroying the object.*

Further proof to this concept can be deduced from the Chayei Adam, who paskens that even in a scenario where there is great exertion involved in saving an item, one does not transgress bal tashchis by letting it go to waste.[2] *Rather, one is considered*

---

1 See *Rashi, Menachos* 81a; *Rambam, Sefer Hamitzvos;* and *Sefer Hachinuch* 529; and others.

2 *Klal* 11, *se'if* 32.

to have "saved" their time and effort. We can apply this here, where, all the more so, the eating of these harmful foods is considered destructive, and throwing them away is saving the person from harm.

Ideally, when one purchases food items, care should be taken to only buy the necessary amount so that no waste will be necessary. One should also be careful when discarding food to wrap it in a bag and throw it out in a respectful manner, as is stated in Shulchan Aruch.[3]

I will end with a berachah—that you should have continued success in teaching proper eating habits that produce health and longevity. Unfortunately, in recent years, there have been those who promote harmful diets, and many get caught in their traps. What they promote is against the Torah's commandment "You shall be very careful to guard your body." I therefore bless your efforts with great success.

Rabbi Yisroel Derbaremdiger

ב"ה

שלום רב ושפעת מרומים לצוות העוסקים במלאכתן באמונה, להורות לרבים הדרך אשר ילכו בה בהתרגלות בסדרי אכילה המועילה לבריאות הגוף והנפש, בשיטה הנקרא "BKCoaching" המפורסם לתהלה ולשבח.

בקשתם ממני לחוות דעתי בכתב בנושא אשר רבים שואלים אודות איסור בל תשחית בזריקת מאכלים הראויים לאכילה לאשפה, במקרה אשר אין באכילתה תועלת, והוא לא מתאים לסדר אכילה בריאה.

באמת, איסור בל תשחית בהשחתת דברים הראויים לשימוש הוא לרוב ראשונים איסור תורה (עי' רש"י מנחות פ"א א' ד"ה ומשני, רמב"ם בספהמ"צ, וחינוך מצוה תקכ"ט ועוד), אך בנידון דידן ברור שמותר לזורקן לאשפה ואף מצוה קעביד, שהרי בגמ' מסכת שבת דף קכ"ט א' מבואר שהתירו לשרוף כלים בכדי להציל מהשחתת הגוף וכלשון הגמ' "בל תשחית דגופא עדיף", והטעם מבואר, דשורש האיסור הוא דדרך התורה

3 See *Orach Chaim*, *siman* 171, which discusses the severity of treating foods properly.

לנצל כל נברא לתכליתו ולצורך תשמישו ולא לגרום איבוד והשחתה לשום חפץ, צא ולמד מיעקב אבינו שחזר בשביל פכים קטנים, אך כל זה הוא כשהוא דרך השחתה ואיבוד אבל באופן שאם יציל את החפץ מאיבוד יושחת עי״ז נפש האדם שהוא תכלית הבריאה, בוודאי בל תשחית דגופא עדיף ולא נקרא כלל השחתת החפץ, וגדולה מזו מצאנו בחיי אדם כלל י״א סל״ב דאף באופן שיש טירחה יתירא בהצלת החפץ אינו עובר בל תשחית דאינו נקרא השחתה אלא הצלת טירחה וזמן, קל וחומר בענינינו שאדרבה האכילה היא ההשחתה והזריקה לאשפה היא ההצלה.

ובוודאי שלכתחילה כשקונים מאכלים צריך ליזהר לקנות רק כמה שצריך כדי שלא יצטרך אח״כ לזרוק לאיבוד, וגם יש ליזהר כשזורקים מאכלים לאשפה לעטפו בשקית ולזרקם בדרך כבוד כמבואר באו״ח סי׳ קע״א חומר איסור ביזוי אוכלין.

ואסיים בברכה, שתזכו להרבות פעלים להפצת המהלך שלכם שמרבה בריאות ומרבה חיים, כי לצערינו הרב לאחרונה רבתה המכשלה ע״י המפיצים שיטות שונות המסגפים את הגוף ומזיקים לבריאות, ורבים נלכדים במצודתן, אך הוא נגד התורה ונשמרתם מאד לנפשותיכם, על כן אמינא לפעולותיכם יישר חילכם להנהיג לאכול בדרך הטוב והבריא, וכלשון החינוך ״ללמד נפשינו לאהוב הטוב והתועלת״ ומסיים ״והחפץ בטוב ושמח בו נפשו בטוב תלין, זה ידוע ומפורסם״.

וע״ז באעה״ח יום י״ג אייר תשפ״ג

ABOUT THE AUTHOR

SINCE 2008, Basya Kovacs has helped thousands of clients reach and maintain their goal weight with her fun and no-nonsense approach. More recently, Basya founded the BKCoaching Center, where she offers private and group coaching. Basya is the host of the very popular podcast *Rise.Shine.Grow*, a weekly source of inspiration, motivation, and entertainment, now streaming on all platforms. In addition, she is the founder of BKSnacking—a line of better-for-you snacks, available in most kosher supermarkets and at bksnacking.com. When not traveling the world, Basya resides in Clifton, New Jersey, with her ever-tolerant husband and five beautiful children.

To book private or group coaching or a speaking engagement, please reach out to Basya at bkcoaching2023@gmail.com.

Visit her website at mybkcoaching.com.